Purchasing Power in Health

Linda Bergthold

PURCHASING
POWER
IN HEALTH

Business, the State, and Health Care Politics

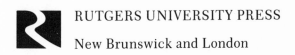

RUTGERS UNIVERSITY PRESS

New Brunswick and London

Library of Congress Cataloging-in-Publication Data

Bergthold, Linda, 1941–
    Purchasing power in health : business, the state, and health care
politics / Linda Bergthold.
      p.   cm.
    Includes bibliographical references.
    ISBN 0-8135-1487-8
    1. Medical care—United States—Cost control.   2. Medical policy—
United States—Business community participation.   3. Medical care—
Political aspects—United States.   I. Title.
RA410.53.B47   1990
338.4'33621'0973—dc20   89-37778
                                                             CIP

British Cataloging-in-Publication information available

For Gary, Lara, Eric, and Alex

Contents

Preface

IT WAS AN unusually hot day for Monterey, California. I had no idea
that the conference session I was about to attend that afternoon in
1982 would give me a book topic. I was just looking for the room
where there was a session on recent Medicaid changes in California.
In that stuffy, hotel conference room, Dr. Leonard Duhl, of the University of California, Berkeley, painted a dynamic picture of social
and political change. Something dramatic had just happened in California health care politics, and I was going to find out more about it.

I was no newcomer to health care politics. I had spent six years in
the 1970s participating in community health planning, learning first-
hand about the futility of health system change through top-down
tinkering. I had been the consumer representative and president of
the local Health Systems Agency, chairperson of endless Certificate
of Need hearings, and a leader of many local advisory groups. Some
of these efforts even produced results. The new psychiatric unit a
few blocks from my home in Santa Cruz was the product of six years
of planning between the public and the private sector, a model of the
effective use of public power.

With the election of Ronald Reagan, I went back to graduate school.
Health planning was dead, and I wanted additional perspective on
change in the health care system. Combining training in political
sociology with a Pew Health Policy fellowship at the University of
California, San Francisco, I was lucky enough to be a student at a
time when the entire health care system was a teacher.

What happened in California in 1982 was a significant new direction in the way the state paid for health care for Medicaid recipients,
accompanied by private-sector changes that allowed corporate pur-

chasers to negotiate with providers on behalf of their employees. How did those structural changes occur? What happened to Robert Alford's "dynamics without change" in the health care system (Alford 1975)? The participation of business representatives in a statewide coalition turned out to be a key factor breaking the provider monopoly over state health policy decisions in California; there was a new political kid on the block. It wasn't just happening in California; it was happening all over the country.

The research reported in this book emerged from a series of questions about the rise of business as an organized political interest in health care politics. Although I realized that labor played an important role, I chose to limit my focus to what business had been doing. Each question I asked required an appropriate research methodology: the "what happened in California and/or Massachusetts" questions led to the case study method, where interviews of key actors and analysis of documents could reconstruct the policy process in its richest detail; the "is this a unique phenomenon or can it be generalized" questions led to secondary and comparative analyses of surveys and documents describing health policy activity at the federal level and in all fifty states.

I had originally selected California as a state case study on the basis of accessibility, cost, and the importance of policy change occurring there in 1982. As the work expanded, I selected Massachusetts because it, too, presented a clear case of business involvement in health policy change within the same time frame as the California changes. Massachusetts also provided political and geographical contrasts to California.

A variation of strategic informant sampling, the "snowball" sample, was used to select informants at state and federal levels. I used a reputational strategy for locating key or strategic actors recommended by knowledgeable observers or selected from lists of participants in a given organization. In the state case studies, business coalitions in each state consisted of key interest group representatives: business, hospitals, physicians, insurers, and government, and in California, labor and senior citizens. I added to that list government bureaucrats, legislators, and academics.

In California, I conducted eighteen face-to-face semistructured interviews and about a dozen telephone interviews; notes from a very generous researcher, Dr. Jerry Briscoe from the University of the Pacific, added fifteen additional informants to the list. In Massachusetts, I interviewed about thirty key actors and sent drafts of the chapter to about thirty additional people for comments. For the study of business participation at the federal level, I relied on interviews with informants who had "been there," plus an analysis of weekly policy bulletins and documents produced by policy think tanks, business associations, and government offices.

My investigation of the participation of business was limited to the period between 1969 and 1988, focusing most of the interviews on events occurring between 1982 and 1988. As a key year for policy change at the state level, I selected 1982 because of changes in federal policy in 1981; however, it became apparent that events leading up to 1982 were important in setting the stage for policy changes in the 1980s, and the years following 1982 were important indicators of the impact of these changes. Thus, I selected 1969 for the beginning of the study because it was the first year of the most recent cycle of corporate intervention in medical care (see Chapter 3).

This research also required investigating all levels of business activity, from local to national. By studying the local level—cities and communities—one learns about individual business or coalition efforts, but most policy decisions are not made at that level. The state level—particularly state level commissions and the legislative arena—can provide a broader picture of the participation of business, but, unless all states are studied, regional variations will confound the explanations. The federal level—national policy-making and legislative bodies—can provide the best window on the way in which the interests of big business mold the formation of policy before it is ever implemented; however, it is difficult to get data on these interactions because they so often occur out of the public eye.

Not all interventions by business led to significant health policy change. Some coalitions and interventions failed to produce any policy change or only symbolic change, and there is no case study here of a significant policy failure. I would advocate such a comparative study in further research.

A multilevel, multimethod research approach avoids the trap of generalizing from a single policy, a single case study, or a single set of actors. I have paid particular attention to the historical context of each policy event in the case studies, the development of certain policies over time, the historical interaction of the political interests, and the consequences of single policy decisions on other policies and interests. By combining several methods (e.g., the case study, historical research, survey analysis), I have tried to broaden this work beyond the policy investigations often reported in the literature by looking at the formation stages of policy, not only the implementation (Stone 1976); examining the interaction of public and private representatives, not only the behavior of private officials (Dahl 1961); and acknowledging the control over resources that big business can command in a community, instead of regarding all actors in the health policy arena as equal in power (Useem 1984; Domhoff 1978).

This research is closest to the concept of a "collaborative exploration" in which the researcher, conscious of her values and biases, makes them explicit. As Rowbottom suggests (probably for a male researcher), "the researcher should take off his shirt and be a participant" (1977:50). Although I do not view this work in the interventionist way Rowbottom might suggest, I do understand that my very choice of topic and approach implies certain values I hold about politics and a democratic society. I believe that certain interests hold more power than others, and it should be clear from my selection of facts and the tone of this book that I admire and respect the role that business leaders have played in challenging provider interests in health care. To admire and understand the business role, however, does not mean that I wish to see business and the state become so dominant that they shut out the other interests. Although much research on business power implies that business is so powerful that the participation of others is futile, I do not believe it, nor do I intend to leave that impression. Despite the unruly nature of participative politics and the difficulty of getting things done when all the actors participate, I still value messy democracy over the available alternatives.

Acknowledgments

As C. WRIGHT MILLS says, "Only by an act of abstraction that unnecessarily violates social reality can we try to freeze some knife-edge moments" (Mills 1959:151). Many people have helped me freeze these moments and interpret what I have seen. Several deserve special mention.

I have been privileged to work closely with two scholars and gentlemen, in the truest sense of the words: Bob Alford was my mentor and colleague at the University of California, Santa Cruz, and is currently chair of the graduate program at City University of New York. Bob directed my dissertation, consulted with me in my first research position at the University of California, San Francisco (UCSF), helped me think through my argument for this book, and encouraged me to "take him on" and carry his work in *Health Care Politics* into the 1980s. Larry Brown is a mentor and colleague, formerly at the University of Michigan and currently head of the Division of Health Administration of the School of Public Health at Columbia University. Larry has been supportive of my work since I was a Pew health policy fellow. He gave up part of his summer in Florida to read the first draft of this book and has given freely of his time and advice as I have struggled to get the manuscript to press.

Other academic colleagues who have contributed to my work include Bill Domhoff, at the University of California, Santa Cruz, a member of my dissertation committee always enthusiastic about my research; Carroll Estes, principal investigator of a research project on posthospital care and the elderly that I directed at the Institute for Health & Aging, UCSF; Phil Lee, director of the Institute for Health Policy Studies at UCSF, whose personal health policy experience provided me with a walking encyclopedia of information about health policy changes at the national level; Leonard Duhl, of the University of California, Berkeley, who started me on my investigation of California's MediCal reform; Bruce Spitz of Brandeis University, whose cachinnations and irreverence kept me honest about my material; Hal Salzman of Boston University, a friend from Santa Cruz and later a crucial informant for the Massachusetts case study; Adam Tachner, a Berkeley graduate, who helped me track down quotes and sources; Alan Sager, of Boston University, whose knowledge of Massachusetts health policy was invaluable; Susan Sherry, leader of the consumer movement in Massachusetts and a key informant on the case study; Deborah Stone of Brandeis University, who read a first draft of the manuscript and whose positive response encouraged me during the long summer of revision; and John T. Dunlop of Harvard University, who opened the door of the Dunlop Group a crack so I could understand how health policy is made behind the scenes.

The policy, provider, and business leaders who are the stars of this book also deserve acknowledgment: Governors Jerry Brown of California and Michael Dukakis of Massachusetts, who provided the context and leadership within which public-private partnerships could succeed; state legislators such as John Garamendi, Willie Brown, and David Roberti in California, and Patricia McGovern, Dan Foley, and Chester Atkins in Massachusetts; provider leaders such as Charles White of the California Hospital Association, David Kinzer and Steve Hegarty of the Massachusetts Hospital Association, Dick Rogen of Blue Cross in Massachusetts, Walter McNerney, former president of Blue Cross and Blue Shield of America, Bernard Tresnowski, its current president, Jim Sammons of the American Medical Association, Jack Light of the California Medical Association, Neil Foley of the Massachusetts Medical Society, Alexander Williams of the American Hospital Association, and David Winston, Reagan's White House "Health Czar," formerly of Blyth Eastman Paine Webber Health Care Funding, Inc., Washington, D.C.

The business leaders are too many to mention here; however, Bill Goldbeck of the Washington Business Group on Health, John Crosier and Nelson Gifford of the Massachusetts Business Roundtable, Bob Lee and Clark Kerr of the California business coalitions, and Nick La Trenta of the Dunlop Group staff and Metropolitan Life Insurance Company, all provided special insight about business and health care politics.

My current employer and friend, Dr. Arnold Milstein, of the Medical Audit Services unit of William M. Mercer, Inc., offered me not only a challenging job and the time and support to finish this book but also a working laboratory in which to test my ideas about the willingness of business to tackle the difficult work of health care cost containment.

My husband Gary deserves the largest share of credit. In our hours of talk about the substance of the book, he helped me think through my argument, edited my sociological jargon, and provided me with a loving and supportive home environment in which to work. Our children, Lara, Eric, and Alex, were proud of me, respectful of my space and time, and fortunately at an age when they were happy to be spending time on their own work and friends. I am proud I seldom shut the door on their soft requests, "Mom, do you have a minute?" Finally, my parents' needs for a health care system more responsive to retirees kept me motivated and writing.

Portions of this book have appeared in the following articles: "Business and the Pushcart Vendors," *International Journal of Health Services* 17, no. 1 (1987): 7–26; "The Business Community as a Promoter of Change," *Business and Health* 3, no. 3 (January/February 1986): 39–41 (reprinted by special permission; copyright 1986, Washington Business Group on Health); and "Crabs in a Bucket: The Politics of Health Care Reform in California," *Journal of Health Politics, Policy and Law* 9, no. 2 (Summer 1984): 203–222 (copyright 1984, Duke University).

Purchasing Power in Health

1

Business and Health Care Politics

HEALTH CARE POLITICS have changed from stalemated "dynamics without change" in the 1960s and 1970s to turbulent "alliances for change" in the 1980s. In the 1960s, there was policy change aplenty but little change in the balance of power among the political interest groups. In the 1980s, "alliances for change"—business alliances with the state; business coalitions with other business; business partnerships with labor; and business federations with providers—have altered the political landscape.[1]

How has health care changed? In the 1960s, health care was still considered a "social good"; in the 1980s, it is regarded by many as a business, and the buyers call the sellers "illness care providers." In the 1960s, health providers railed against state intervention as socialized medicine; in 1983, the passage of prospective payment, one of the most intrusive regulatory schemes to be implemented in the past twenty years, was hailed as "procompetition," and the state was called a "prudent purchaser" of care.[2] In the 1960s, doctors could be individual entrepreneurs or "pushcart vendors," without being drawn into the "age of supermarkets," represented by the multihospital systems and preferred provider networks. Doctors were firmly in charge of health policy decisions in the 1960s, as they shaped the "interior of reform" that was called Medicare.[3] Now they complain about competing with each other like "crabs in a bucket," put there by both public and private purchasers of care.[4]

Community hospitals in the 1960s were proudly embedded in community life. In the 1980s, hospital care is often provided by major corporations, and the popular television show "St. Elsewhere" even dramatized the acquisition of a public hospital by a multinational corporation. In the 1960s policymakers talked about access to care for the poor and the elderly; the discussions of the 1980s have been focused almost exclusively on the cost of care, with occasional sidebars on quality and access. In the 1960s, business leaders were passive observers of the Medicare debate; in the 1980s they have been more aggressive participants in health care politics at all levels.

Times have changed, and they have changed substantially. What accounts for these changes?

I argue that business may well be the "fat kid on the seesaw" that has tipped the balance in health care politics.[5] This book tells the story of a period of almost two decades (1969–1988) when business became actively involved in health care politics; it describes the participation of business in health policy formation, the organizations that business mobilized to promote its interests, and the types of policies that business interests have promoted. What started as a solo trumpet call for business involvement by Robert Finch, Richard Nixon's secretary of health, education, and welfare in 1969, becomes an entire brass band by the end of the 1980s.[6]

The term "business" (or "corporate") as used in the book describes the activities and the economic interests of big business. Most corporations involved in the formulation of policy, at either the state or federal level, are of the Fortune 500 variety, and the organizations that express business interests are dominated, in either leadership or membership, by big business interests. Although large and important corporate interests are involved in the production and financing of medical care services, the term "business" as used in this book will refer to *employers* as *purchasers* of medical care services for their employees.[7]

Business representatives, in this purchaser role, have intervened in the health policy debate several times in the past fifty years. The intensity of business political participation increased in the 1970s as the rising costs of employee health premiums began noticeably to affect company profits. For example, between 1970 and 1982, the nominal growth in the GNP was 208 percent; U.S. health expenditures increased 332 percent, but employer health benefit expenditures increased 700 percent.[8] In 1976, the average company spent about 5 percent of its payroll on health benefits; in 1988 it had almost doubled to 9.7 percent.[9] In 1984, the Big Three auto companies alone spent $3.5 billion for health care. That was more than each of thirty-two states collected in taxes and spent in that year.[10] The increasing costs of health care were going straight to the bottom line of most major American corporations, and the amount was staggering.

Business responded to these increasing costs by restructuring company health benefit packages and asking employees to share in these costs. Business also became organized and politically involved. The Business Roundtable (BR), a national association of Fortune 500 companies, formed the Washington Business Group on Health (WBGH) in the mid-1970s to monitor and tackle health care cost issues. In 1982 only twenty-five business coalitions existed across the country to address issues of containing health care cost. By 1988, of the 175 active coalitions in forty-six states, 45 percent characterized themselves as "employer-only."[11]

Throughout the 1970s and 1980s, business leaders have been increasingly visible in the halls of state capitols, at commissions, task force tables, and legislative hearings, as they have attempted to bring some rationality and business principles to bear on the frustrating and sometimes "dirty project" of health care cost containment.[12]

First, business began to talk about the problem:

• In 1973 a representative of big business to the Committee for Economic Development (CED), a national corporate study group, commented, "Our health care industry is the only major industry that has not had to submit to the discipline of either the marketplace or of public regulation. As a result, the industry has inadequate cost-control mechanisms, and the rate of rise in health care costs has far outstripped that of any other segment of our economy."[13]

• In 1984, in testimony before the Joint Economic Committee of Congress, Joseph Califano, former secretary of health and human services for President Carter and a current director of Chrysler Corporation, commented, "This month for the first time in our history, Americans are spending more than $1 billion a day on health care. . . . This year Chrysler will have to sell 70,000 vehicles just to pay for its health care bills. . . . True reductions in cost will come only from fundamental changes in the way we deliver and pay for health care . . . and concerted action by all the players."[14]

• By 1986, the executive director of the Massachusetts Roundtable was saying, "The easy part of health care cost containment is now behind us and the real tough part is ahead. . . . At some point parochial interests have to be set aside and people have to worry about the whole system. . . . If the industry's leaders do not get together and talk about this problem, then the budget builders in the government and the private sector will create situations to force them to deal with it."[15]

Business also began to do something about the problem, although not all these interventions produced sustained cost containment:

• Nelson Gifford, the chief executive officer (CEO) of Dennison Manufacturing Company in Massachusetts, frustrated by a stalemated public cost containment debate, identified who was powerful and invited them to join him in his private offices in Waltham in 1982. Policy was made, as one participant noted, "like a party at your house." This private coalition forged a regulatory policy solution outside the legislature that resulted in the passage of hospital cost containment legislation. By the end of the second year after the legislation was passed, total hospital costs had increased only 6.2 percent in Massachusetts, and increases in health insurance premiums were the lowest in a decade.[16]

• In 1984, Sperry, Motorola, and Garrett corporation executives in Arizona, angry because hospital administrators were flying high in corporate jets while hospital costs to business soared even higher, took their message about cost containment to the people through a statewide initiative process because the legislature would not respond quickly enough. Even though the initiative lost, the business community became a permanent and active participant in the political process.

• The Dexter Corporation's president, Worth Loomis, told a conference of governors in 1984 that his company's health care costs were the third highest single item of costs, following only raw materials and direct compensation. These costs, which had been increasing by 15 to 20 percent a year, decreased by 10.5 percent during the first quarter of 1984 and per employee costs dropped by 13.5 percent through an aggressive company cost-containment effort. Loomis commented, "We employers, whether state, municipal, nonprofit or private, have a choice of committing suicide or seeing to it that provider behavior is substantially altered."[17]

• In 1984, a small but determined coterie of Iowa business representatives sat in the deserted halls of the state capitol one midnight waiting to buttonhole legislators on their way out of a hearing on health insurance changes. Hospital use in Iowa was 18 percent over the national average, and employers were ready to use "the clout that comes with paying the bill."[18]

• Bob Lee, the vice president of Plantronics in California, obtained state data on hospital costs in his plant's town in 1988 and took the printouts to his negotiating session with hospital administrators. His knowledge of their costs forced them to give him a substantial discount for his employees. These negotiations and other cost-containment activities helped bring Plantronics's cost per employee down to about $1,500 per employee per year, lower than the national average.[19]

• Edward Hennessy, CEO of Allied-Signal Corporation, commented in *The Wall Street Journal* in 1988, "Companies . . . need to start making better use of their bargaining power . . . to make U.S. industry a customer that has to be reckoned with in the healthcare marketplace. We must persuade providers to take a seat beside us on the cost containment bandwagon." Allied's health care costs, twice as high as the medical care consumer price index (CPI) in the early 1980s, had moderated in the mid-1980s because of a host of internal company cost-containment strategies. By 1987, however, their costs soared 39 percent in one year, sending Allied into their communities all over the country to modify the delivery system. An alliance with one insurer, CIGNA corporation, and a proactive health maintenance organization enrollment strategy, predicted savings of $200 million between 1987 and 1990.[20]

• The president of the Washington Business Group on Health said in 1984, "The biggest educational step has not been in dealing with business about government, but in breaking business away from the providers. . . . We have broken down the myths that kept business as a passive purchaser, and we have made them aggressive buyers."[21]

Business Interventions for Change

To explain how business became involved at the local, state, and federal levels, I have highlighted three types of business interventions:

1. Business organized specific *institutional mechanisms* for change, such as coalitions, associations, and lobbying groups. "Organization is itself a mobilization of bias in preparation for action."[22] Chapter 3 explains the forces that propelled business into political activity in the 1970s through a review of the American economic and political context and a media scan of major business and health journals of the 1970s and 1980s. Chapter 4 describes five specific institutional mechanisms for change that business created or used to promote its message: the Chamber of Commerce of the U.S. and its health policy committee; the Business Group on Health; the Dunlop Group of Six, an informal policy group consisting of the leadership of the six major stakeholders in health care politics (hospitals, insurers, Blue Cross, physicians, business, and labor); and business and health coalitions around the country.

2. The *business advisory role* to state and federal governments, such as policy committees in Washington and the formation of the Dunlop Group of Six, emerged in health policy. Chapter 4 describes the work of business in the Dunlop Group of Six, and Chapter 5 provides the federal context for state-level policy change in the early 1980s. The ideology of policy change and the advisory role that business played in key national committees and commissions demonstrate another level of business participation and interaction with the state.

3. The direct *legislative participation* of business leaders at the state level, such as the participation of business in the Roberti Coalition in Cal-

ifornia and the Health Care Coalition in Massachusetts, was initiated. Chapters 6 and 7 are two state case studies of business activity in commissions and legislative advocacy. These chapters describe two different contexts in which business power was exercised and demonstrate different degrees of concentration of business power. In both states, business was brought into the policy process by the state, and business interests and state power in alliance were able to help break the provider grip on the policy process and promote substantial policy change. Chapter 8 compares the political and economic contexts in both states and explains the different levels of business participation and policy outcomes. Chapter 9 gives an overview of business participation and policy change in all fifty states.

I chose these three types of business interventions for their diversity, political significance, and researchability.[23] The diversity of settings in which business leaders have attempted to change policy ranges from individual companies to local coalitions to national advisory committees. The state case studies and the fifty state chapter were included because, by all accounts, something politically significant had happened in California and Massachusetts in 1982, and, as it turned out, this type of change was happening all over the country. All the interventions described in this book had to be researchable, in the sense that I was able to interview key actors, locate documents and articles describing these events, or observe events personally. Clearly, many people acted and made decisions in settings inaccessible to me or by actors with whom I could not or did not make contact. I have dealt with these black holes of information by sending drafts of my work to almost every person whom I interviewed, and some whom I did not, to test my descriptions and conclusions against their perceptions.

The Parameters of the Business Power Debate

When you write about business power, you steer a perilous course between the Scylla of beliefs about business unity and the Charybdis of ideas about business fragmentation. To help explain where I stand in this debate, I present the following statements about business power, based on my own ideas as well as my research.

• Business is *not* unified; it is fragmented. However, business interests are neither too fragmented to act politically at all nor so powerful and organized that whenever they choose to participate they have whatever impact they intend.[24] "Large corporations through their ability to expand, contract, or simply redefine employment opportunities, productive capacity, and other of society's resources have become among the most important of these large scale institutions. . . . When these corporations are feuding and atomized, their political impact tends to be inconsistent, at times contradictory, and thus neutralized. When less divided and better organized for collective action, however, they can be very effective in finding and promoting their shared concerns."[25] I acknowledge the systemic and class-based power of business, but the data presented here focus on the application of business power in discrete political situations, and thus the diversity of business interests is often more apparent than potential or actual unity.

● The relationship of business and state power is complex, interactive, and central to the discussion in this book because the state is the central arena in which the process of politics unfolds. It makes no sense to talk about business power in policy formation without also discussing the relationship of business and the state. Successful alliances between business and the state, however, can occur only under certain conditions: a perceived policy crisis, relatively united interest groups, and a political context that encourages and allows this fusion of power. Given the fragmented nature of American politics, it should not be surprising that this type of alliance does not occur more often. This book offers several instances in which business and the state have worked together as purchasers of health care to effect policy reform.

● Business has the power to initiate policy change and ally itself with other interests. "The business sector cannot, of course, change the system singlehandedly. It can, however, be instrumental in bringing about needed changes in the reimbursement system by using its purchasing-power muscle and forging a coalition of legislators, producers, and insurers to support necessary legislation."[26] This does not mean that business will always initiate change; only that it has the power to do so, and when it forms alliances with other interests, such as the state, the combined purchasing power of both sectors can be sufficient to force change on a resistant system.

● Not all business leaders participate in political activity; in fact, only a few CEOs of companies have been involved in health care politics over the years. More commonly, vice presidents of personnel or human resources have been designated to communicate the corporate message.[27] However, the larger the firm, the more likely it is that the chief officer will be aware of the political issues. "The head of a big business firm has a great potential for influencing public policy in the direction which he prefers."[28] Even though CEOs placed health care at a level of four or five on a scale of one hundred in the early 1980s, the importance of cost containment has certainly inched up since then. Most

CEOs now know that health care costs are important and can be partially controlled within their own corporations.

• Business is powerful whether it participates or not. Business usually gets politically involved because business needs are not being met through the policy process. "Business organised little to protect its collective interests in the USA in the 1950s because its collective interests were little challenged."[29] Even though business participation in health policy leveled off in the mid-1980s, it is likely to increase or take new forms in the 1990s as individual company strategies and even purchaser alliances ultimately fail to bring health care costs under control. Business will begin participating to the degree its interests are further challenged by rising costs because its effectiveness in controlling health care costs will be diminished by business fragmentation and the powerful contradictions between business as purchaser and as provider of health care.

• When business participates, it does *not* win every policy battle. The participation, even by dominant business firms, does not automatically translate into situational political influence or successful policy outcomes. Business may be powerful at societal levels, but it cannot always translate its market power into concrete legislative outcomes. The fact that business lost in Pennsylvania in 1982, when the Business Council failed to produce the legislative change it promoted that year, does not mean business is weak. By 1988, business interests in Pennsylvania had reorganized, successfully challenged the providers, and gained passage of some of their legislative objectives.

• Even when aroused to awareness, there are many barriers to corporate action. Business leaders tend to react to crisis rather than plan ahead to avoid it. Most business leaders tire easily of the amount of hassling, meeting, reading, and confronting it takes to be an effective agent in health care cost containment. In addition, it is often personally unpleasant to exercise purchasing power. Hospital administrators frown when business trustees become too critical of hospital plans for expansion, and doctors refuse to talk to them at the country club. Health care politics involves plenty of political and personal risks.

Despite the barriers to action, the complexity of the issues, the lack of unity among business sectors, the considerable action taken is all the more remarkable. In the next chapters I will describe the forces that drove business leaders to overcome their reticence about health care politics and confront problems of health care cost and quality in their own companies and communities. I believe that American business, in alliance with the state and other interests, has significantly contributed to health policy in the past twenty years. Understanding that contribution can help us predict likely business reactions in the next few decades and the likely directions of the health care industry in response.

2

Power, Policy, and Politics

THREE INTERRELATED THEMES are woven throughout this book: *power, policy,* and *politics.* Each theme requires answering key questions. Power: Of what does the power of business consist? Under what conditions can business most successfully exercise its power? What explains the success or failure of business when it chooses to act politically in health care? Policy: What is the policy impact of business participation? What policies are consistent with business interests? Politics: What explains the emergence of business as a political actor? What are the consequences of alliances between business and the state?

It is almost impossible to separate these themes and questions from one another. For example, when people ask about business power, they inevitably learn about the policies business promotes. When they investigate the policy process, they learn about business as a political actor. And the question of the alliance of business with the state is linked at the most fundamental level to all three themes of business power, policy process, and politics of health care. The evidence presented in this book cannot answer all the questions raised. It can only highlight key issues, identify some bodies of theory that speak to these issues, and locate questions within these powerful and unresolved debates.

Power

"The definition of the alternatives is the supreme instrument of power; ... he who determines what politics is about runs the country, because the definition of the alternatives is the choice of conflicts, and the choice of conflicts allocates power."

E. E. Schattschneider, *The Semi-Sovereign People*

In order to understand under what conditions business power can be most successfully exercised, one must look more closely at the meaning of power. Several social science traditions attempt to define levels of power. The "one-dimensional" approach has been most commonly associated with pluralist political science researchers such as Robert Dahl and Nelson Polsby.[1] This approach regards power as the ability of A to exercise power over B to get B to do something B would not ordinarily do. Pluralists generally conduct behavioral studies of decision-making power by political actors and ask who wins, who loses, and who participates. Pluralists observe that the system may be biased toward one group or another, but they believe that the political system balances these biases and that the state intervenes to protect all interests equally. Pluralists do not usually investigate the way in which the political agenda is controlled by one group or another or how power might be exercised to prevent an issue from ever being considered.

A pluralist view of business power would regard that power as predominantly situational and almost solely dependent on economic cycles; that is, when business begins to lose too much money it will enter the policy arena and attempt to influence policies inimical to its interests. Business leadership is more important than the organizations that business constructs to represent its interests. In the game of legislation, business wins some and loses some. Business might cooperate with government in public-private partnerships, but business power is seldom seen as dominant in forming the policy agenda.

A pluralist recognizes business power and may decry its growth and penetration in American political life; however, most pluralists believe that the electoral process can offset the undue exercise of that power. Charles Lindblom's disquieting final paragraph in *Politics and Markets* reflects the ambivalence of the pluralist study of business power: "It has been a curious feature of democratic thought that it has not faced up to the private corporation as a peculiar organization in an ostensible democracy.... Enormously large, rich in resources, the big corporations, we have seen, command more resources than do most government units. ...The large private corporation fits oddly into democratic theory and vision. Indeed, it does not fit."[2]

When pluralists point to business losses in a political situation or to the varying levels of effectiveness of business participation as examples where business is just another interest, albeit a powerful one, they sometimes fail to separate out the different levels of business power and their appropriate units of analysis. Business possesses market- or class-based power through its ownership and control of production resources in a community or jurisdiction; business demonstrates structural power through its mobilization of organizations and its access to the policy formation process; and finally business has situational power through business leadership and influence in the political arena. In attempting to define business power, it is important to identify what level of business power is being exercised and what type of evidence appropriately indicates that level of power. The case study chapters offer examples of exercising all three levels of business power but emphasize the structural or organizational power of business.[3]

The "two-dimensional" approach to power is most closely associated with Peter Bachrach and Morton Baratz, although their work builds on earlier work done by E. E. Schattschneider, who studied the organized, special interest group system he calls the "pressure system."[4] In the view of Bachrach and Baratz, power is demonstrated not only in decisions made but also in decisions not made and in the exclusion of some groups from participation in the political process. Bachrach and Baratz are interested in the way bias is mobilized, and their work analyzes the dominant values, myths, and procedures of the political game. An example of a study of nondecision is the work of Matthew Crenson on the role of U.S. Steel in preventing certain air pollution policies from being considered in Gary, Indiana.[5]

A two-dimensional view of business power would investigate the way business elites controlled and occasionally dominated the agenda formation process in health in certain states in the 1980s. When policies did not produce the needed changes, as happened in the 1970s with a failed "voluntary effort" by hospitals to control costs, business was compelled to participate more actively in the policy formation process. The two-dimensional view, with its emphasis on exclusion as well as inclusion of political groups, would help to explain why labor and sometimes even physicians were excluded from the policy formation process in Massachusetts, for example.

The most abstract view of power, the "three-dimensional" approach, is also the most difficult to investigate through a case study method. This approach is associated with Steven Lukes, who regards power as a situation in which A exercises power over B in a manner contrary to B's interests. This approach describes the way A molds B's interests and prevents conflict from ever occurring.[6] Among the works that successfully show ways in which power can be exercised through manipulating symbols and ideology is John Gaventa's *Power and Powerlessness,* an analysis of the conditions that fostered quiescence but finally rebellion within a powerless group in an Appalachian valley.[7]

Although it would have been helpful to include more material on the way business interests prevented issues from being placed on the legislative agenda or controlled the issues being considered and the actors who could participate, there are some examples of this approach in the case study chapters. Lukes's analysis makes observers aware of the symbolic importance of holding the Massachusetts coalition meetings in the offices of the Business Roundtable or the way state legislators in California used the affection of special interests for the "competitive" approach to policy change to implement a stronger system of state intervention.

Furthermore, the three-dimensional approach to the study of power helps explain how the power of business can often deny and obfuscate issues to those participating in the policy process. Few participants will acknowledge the power of business to control the policy agenda, least of all business representatives themselves. As one Massachusetts legislative assistant noted when asked to comment on the power of business in that state, "I'm not sure there are many legislators who want to put a gun near their head and find out how real the power of business is."[8]

Another aspect of power is its relationship to participation. Does participation always lead to power? Does power require participation? Or might power be exercised without any visible political participation at all? Robert Alford and Roger Friedland explore several relationships between power and participation that are relevant to these case studies: (1) participation without power, that is, symbolic participation; (2) power without participation, that is, systemic power; and (3) power with participation, that is, structural power.[9] These concepts of power and participation permit a more complex view of the role of business in policy formation. It is not enough to know who wins or loses in a given legislative battle. The power of business can be demonstrated at several levels simultaneously. What type of power does business have in the Alford and Friedland schema?

Participation without power—symbolic participation—is sometimes characteristic of the outcomes of some commissions and committees described in this book. In the late 1970s and early 1980s, health care costs were substantially higher than other costs of doing business. Given the real crisis in rising health care costs, one might expect structural changes in the way health care was purchased, financed, and delivered. Indeed, many changes in the 1980s (e.g., prospective payment, contracting, balanced billing of physicians, etc.) can be characterized as changes altering fundamental power relationships between interest groups. However, there have also been a multitude of more symbolic attempts to solve these policy problems. The emergence of statewide commissions that usually included representatives of public and private purchasers, producers, or providers, and, occasionally, token representatives of consumers and underserved groups, can indicate symbolic politics when the policy solutions proposed neither change the distribution of resources nor lower costs.

Alford and Friedland marshal evidence to demonstrate convincingly that social class is highly correlated with participation but that political participation itself is not highly correlated with changes in expenditure at either the state or local level. Then why would the poor and the under-represented bother participating if resources and power relationships remain unchanged? Alford and Friedland argue that the state often incorporates leaders of the poor into programs using the ideology of "citizen participation," even though there is little evidence that this participation produces policy change. Furthermore, even if individuals do gain something from citizen participation, their participation is limited by the tables to which they are invited.[10]

In the Massachusetts case study (Chapter 7), consumer and labor members were kept out of the private coalition negotiations over health policy change in 1982 but finally invited to participate in the commissions after 1985. Similarly, in California (Chapter 6), consumers and labor were members of the public, state-initiated Roberti Coalition, but they were not involved in the behind-the-scenes legislative maneuvering and state-level lobbying. Because resources are rarely controlled at the local level, allowing the powerless to participate at the local level will seldom substantially challenge the dominant interests, whose power and economic organization are located elsewhere.

Power without participation—systemic power—can be seen in the relationship between economic development at the local or state level and the participation of dominant economic interests. "The fiscal capacity of all units of government is contingent upon the locational, production and investment decisions of increasingly concentrated corporations."[11] Paul Starr, author of *The Social Transformation of American Medicine*, notes the difference between what he calls the market or "structural" power of business and professional power:

The medical profession does not have the same basis of power as large corporations. Private capital is not simply one of several interest groups in society; the economy and hence the government's own tax revenues depend on "business confidence." Hence business confidence generally acts as a constraint on policy without businessmen ever having to lobby on behalf of their interests as a class. If government threatens to undermine business confidence, it jeopardizes its own stability by bringing about a reduction in investment and a general economic crisis, with rising unemployment and lower tax revenues. The medical profession clearly does not have this degree of "structural power."[12]

To sustain its systemic or market power, business does not always have to participate politically. If the fiscal viability of local and state programs depends on the impact of those programs on dominant economic interests, and if those interests do not always have to participate politically to demonstrate or exercise power, then it follows that business interests may not perceive a need to participate and that the state will find it necessary to organize them at times. Their political participation will become, under those conditions, a consequence, not a cause of their power.

The potential power of business and the state, in alliance, allows me to discuss the third relationship between power and participation. Power with participation—what Alford and Friedland term *structural* power"—"refers to the ways in which the particular organization of political authority . . . differentially affects the level and effectiveness of political participation of different social groups. The structure of the state intervenes between participation and power."[13] In both California and Massachusetts in the early 1980s, state officials found it expedient and necessary to organize private business interests. Evidence in later chapters shows that public and private purchaser interests, when combined in strategic alliance, do have the potential to bring about substantial structural change in the health care system. This is "power with participation."

An example of the exercise of power with participation is the formation of strategic alliances between business and the state. The participation of business in public-private sector commissions is neither recent nor limited to the health policy arena. However, it has been largely a symbolic endeavor in health care politics of past years, and business interests have not participated to the degree or intensity they did in the early 1980s. In the short period between 1982 and 1984, at least thirty states had organized state-level commissions to address issues of health care cost containment, and business participated in many of these commissions.[14]

Some have regarded these public-private alliances as evidence for a pluralist theory of politics, in which the state is regarded as a neutral referee between competing groups, with little independent interests of its own. The more groups that participate in the political process, the more competition is assumed to exist. Others have suggested that the interaction of business representatives with producers and state interests is a form of "quasi," "middle-level," or "incipient" corporatism, in the sense of the European model of bargaining and planning between the state, producer, and purchaser interests.[15] Streeck and Schmitter have described corporatism as referring to "two different but interrelated dimensions of interest politics: the way in which group interests in a society are organized and the way in which they are integrated into the policy process so as to make for better accommodation of interest conflicts."[16] Yet the irreconcilable differences between the European and American political contexts, the weakness of the American state, the lack of consensus about social policy, and the inability of the American labor movement to participate equally with other interests are all considerable barriers to corporatist arrangements in this country.[17]

Professor Lawrence Brown notes that the appeal of a corporatist explanation for political bargaining in the American context lies in its "heuristic powers and the hypotheses to which it points, not in its descriptive accuracy."[18] He then describes three types of corporatist interventions in American health care politics that have involved "government-group" relations since the enactment of Medicare: "consensual corporatism" (1965–1972) attempted to rationalize and control health care costs through strategies such as the delegation of power and administrative function to insurance intermediaries; "inverted corporatism" (1972–1977) centralized review and control over the Medicare program, not in Washington, D.C., but in hundreds of state and local entities; and finally, "technocratic corporatism" (1977–present), provides a policy of reorganization, improved data, and national limits on hospital revenues and capital spending.

The questions remain. What theory best explains all the public-private interactions over health policy that occurred at the state level in the early and middle 1980s? Was there a significant state presence in the policy process? A two-way policy implementation process in which the battle over policy formation and implementation was controlled by powerful interest organizations rather than courts or state agencies? And was there occasionally a mobilization of interests reminiscent of the "peak associations" that bargain for political power in the European context? The case study material will help answer some of these questions.

In fact, pluralism and corporatism need not be rival explanations of the political process; instead, they should be regarded as two points on a continuum of political events and groups, measuring the access to power and the role of various groups in specific political situations.[19] The reality of fragmented American politics demands different questions about the contrasts between pluralist and corporatist explanations of the state: one must ask not whether the state is neutral, whether the public and private are separate spheres, whether one is more powerful than the other, or how many groups participating in the political process constitute pluralist competition; but rather one must question under what conditions organized groups are integrated into policy formation, how much competition and concentration of power exists in a given situation, and what are the consequences of a fusion of state and business power, however temporary or fragile, on the process and substance of health policy formation.[20]

Policy

"Making policy is inescapably and properly a political project, one undertaken in the unsettling foreknowledge that although there are endless social transitions to be mediated, there are no right answers to discover or learn."

Lawrence Brown, *Politics and Health Care Organization*

The second theme of this book is the relationship of business participation to the policy-making process in health. What impact has business had, if any, on the policy process and on the substance of health policy? Business interests have helped to change the policy formation process in several ways: business has participated in setting the policy agenda and has encouraged policies consistent with its interests; in some cases, business has changed the rules of the public policy process so they are consistent with private decision-making and negotiation modes; and, in other cases, the public, consumer interest has been made equivalent to purchaser interests.

What is "policy"?[21] Although policy and politics are closely related and in some languages the two words are not even differentiated, I will define policy as the British social scientist Jenkins does. Policy is synonymous with decisions; patterns of decisions over time constitute policy; policy decisions are taken by political actors; policies are about both means and ends; and policies depend upon real situations and feasible projects.[22]

Setting the Policy Agenda: "Setting the agenda is the vital first step of policy formation, which often establishes the parameters for everything that follows. If business misses the real start of the process, it automatically reduces its effectiveness."[23] What role did business play in the agenda formation in the early 1980s? Evidence in later chapters shows the work of the Business Roundtable and the Washington Business Group on Health as well as participation of a few powerful business leaders at the state level and on key Reagan administration policy committees, business interests in the Dunlop Group of Six, and to a lesser extent of the Chamber of Commerce of the U.S. and the National Association of Manufacturers. The presence and visibility of a few key business representatives usually indicate a larger network of business elites who are aware of the policy agenda being developed.

The policy agenda supported by business throughout the 1970s and the early 1980s was pragmatic. Even though President Reagan's administration was proposing a narrowly defined, highly ideological, "market" approach to health care reform in 1981, big business supported the policy proposals they hoped would bring down health care costs. During the 1970s, business had supported alternative delivery systems such as health maintenance organizations (HMOs) and the "voluntary effort" by hospitals, neither of which had affected the rising cost of health care. By the early 1980s, there was evidence that regulatory approaches such as rate-setting for hospital charges in New Jersey and New York could hold down health care costs. In California, business supported regulation before turning to a competitive solution; in Massachusetts, business supported a regulatory solution in 1982 but was promoting more competition by 1988.

The choice of policy strategies by business also depended on the relative strength of labor and the state at the location of policy decisions. In the fifty states, and particularly in those states where labor was strong, such as Michigan, Ohio, or Illinois, more regulatory strategies were selected. At the national level, where labor representation was relatively weak and business input strong, the market strategy of the Reagan administration was stronger. Although not every aspect of Reagan's market ideology benefited every sector of business (particularly the proposed "tax cap" on employer paid benefits), and although there were strategic conflicts within and between various sectors of business over which policies to support or oppose, the major policy direction in the early 1980s was consistent with large purchaser interests in ways that will be described more fully in Chapters 5 and 9.

Business and the policy process: Business did not play a dominant role in all thirty states that formed cost-containment commissions in the 1980s; but business participated much more frequently than labor, and business became a permanent part of the policy process in health through this participation. Few statewide commissions were formed without including representatives of key business organizations. By participating so actively and visibly at the public level, business also introduced changes in the policy process itself. Massachusetts is probably the most extreme case, where business leadership actually took the public policy process out of the legislature and forged a solution in private coalition negotiations. As one participant commented, "Public policy development is different from business decision making. The Chapter 372 policy changes [the Massachusetts legislation] occurred because Gifford [the Health Task Force chairman] made it a business decision making process not a public policy process."[24]

In other states, business participated in a public process but often carried out a private process of lobbying and influence more compatible with private-sector decision making. Depending on the context and the power of business in a given state, business participation could and did lead to a change in the policy process. How is this process different from policy-making processes previously controlled by the state? Although policy decisions have almost always been made in private and ratified in public, at least in the past there have been a variety of structures for participation, symbolic or otherwise (e.g., community action program councils; health systems agencies; certificate of need hearings). Policy alternatives and criteria for negotiation have been set, if not completely by the state, usually with strong state representation, and participation was available to a wide range of stakeholders in the policy process.

In the 1980s, with business playing such a dominant role, the public process might have included labor, consumers, and minorities at the policy table had there been one, but they were not invited to the back rooms and did not have the type of access to public officials that business and the providers had. In some cases, such as Massachusetts in the early 1980s, business purchaser interests were simply identified as synonymous with the public or consumer interest without challenge or discussion. Some observers doubted whether business purchasers could fairly represent all consumer interests.

Politics

"Politics, like religion, love, and the arts, is a theme that men cannot leave alone: not in their behavior, nor in their talk, nor in their writing of history."

Murray Edelman, *The Symbolic Uses of Politics*

This book is about health care politics and the way in which business has come to be a regular and powerful participant at all levels where health policy is made and carried out. What explains the emergence of business as a political actor? Although business has been active at several other periods in the twentieth century, a number of macrolevel issues propelled business leaders to take action about health care costs beginning in the early 1970s: the economic recession of that decade, the seemingly uncontrollable increases in health care costs and the effect of those costs on profit margins, and state policy actions and decisions, including generally increased government regulation. Microissues such as individual firm costs, location, dependence and type of firms in the community, and availability of business leadership also contributed to business participation.

Previous research on health care politics has taken as given the list of participants, their political power, and the fact that when some participants win the others must lose. Physicians are almost always characterized as being dominant and having the most power, followed by hospitals and insurers. The state is generally not included or described as an interest in the same way. Does the evidence in this book always demonstrate increased business participation and power accompanied by decreased power for the other interests? Or can an exercise of power by business result in the increased participation and power of the other interests, including the state?

Studies of health care politics have been surprisingly scant in the past twenty years. Alford has commented, "Strange as it may seem, there are relatively few studies of the politics of health care policy. As recently as 1966 Herbert Kaufman could review major treatises in public health and conclude that none contained more than a passing reference to politics."[25] Even Theodore Marmor, who twenty-five years ago wrote the seminal health care politics book, *The Politics of Medicare*, comments on the lack of innovative ideas in health care politics. "We are living with the debris of the reform mentality of the 1970s."[26] Since the mid-1970s, a few books have been published about health care politics, including Paul Starr's *The Social Transformation of American Medicine*. Most of these books refer to Alford's work, but not even Starr has put forth an adequate alternative to Alford's description of health care interests as "professional monopolists," "corporate rationalizers," and "equal health advocates."[27]

Although *Health Care Politics* has made a substantial contribution to understanding the health care system, several points in Alford's book are worthy of challenge as one tries to understand the participation of business in health care politics in the 1980s. First, he reformulates the conventional idea of "interest groups" into broader categories defined as "structural interests." These interests are not specifically defined (and, as Starr points out, are almost metaphysical in the abstractness of their definition) but described as "more than potential interest groups" because they "either do not have to be organized in order to have their interests served or cannot be organized without great difficulty."[28] There are three types of structural interests: dominant, challenging, and repressed. Dominant interests are those "served by the structure of social, economic and political institutions as they exist at any given time. . . . The interests do not continuously have to organize and act to defend their interests; other institutions do that for them." Challenging structural interests are "those being created by the changing structure of society." In the latter category, Alford places the "corporate rationalizers" mentioned above. Repressed interests are those community and minority interests not served by social institutions and political groups who must muster extraordinary energy and effort to participate in the political process.

Alford did not include business representatives as part of the corporate rationalizer structural interest, not did he anticipate the increasingly dominant role that business representatives of large corporations would play at the local, state, and national level in the 1980s. Does the addition of business representatives to the line-up of corporate rationalizers alter the balance of power in the system? Does it make any sense to include business in the same category as hospital representatives? What about insurers? Within Alford's framework, the corporate rationalizers were already attempting to contradict and challenge the fundamental interests of professional monopolists, but he believed that the conflicts engendered by these challenges would be "contained within an institutional frame-work which prevents corporate rationalization from generating enough social power truly to integrate and coordinate health care."

Whether business and the corporate rationalizers have generated enough power to integrate or coordinate health care is not the subject of this book; that policy study would require collecting different data. Whether the goal of coordination should be or is the major criterion by which social change should be measured is also not within this book's scope, although it is the criterion used by what Alford calls "bureaucratic reformers." However, the addition of business as a political actor to the structural interest of corporate rationalization does suggest that the dominance of physician monopolists is no longer a given in health care politics.

Alford also maintained that no reform efforts would seriously damage "any interests." However, several antitrust decisions have challenged this prediction, the first of which occurred in 1975, mandating competition in the provision of professional services. Physician power has been de-creased as a consequence of following Federal Trade Commission (FTC) decisions: consumers deserve an increased flow of information; physi-cians may advertise under restricted conditions; companies may contract with groups of physicians; individual physicians may enter into contracts for the practice of medicine; and physicians are prevented from restrict-ing the practice of chiropractors and osteopaths. State court decisions have upheld both the removal of "freedom of choice" provisions from state law to allow the growth of preferred provider organizations and the ban on "balanced billing" in Massachusetts, prohibiting physicians from charging more than Medicare will pay them.

These legal challenges to physician authority, along with the increased corporatization and privatization of health care throughout the past two decades, indicate an increase in power for the rationalizers—public and private purchasers—who have supported these changes.[29] The world of health care politics has changed considerably since physicians and hospi-tals controlled health policy-making in the 1960s. This book will demon-strate some ways in which the previously dominant "professional monopolists" (i.e., physicians) have lost both structural and situational power in the political arena. The "corporate rationalizers" (i.e., hospital administrators, medical schools, government health planners, public health agencies and researchers, and business representatives) have be-come more than challenging interests, and I offer evidence here to test that earlier prediction.

To claim that business alone has changed the health care system or the substance of health policy, however, would be to claim much more than the evidence can support. Nevertheless, business has been propelled into active political participation in health policy for various economic and political reasons, and, once involved, it has often played a dominant policy role in structuring both the policy process and its outcomes. When the market power of business purchasers joins the legal power of the state, in the context of choices defined by standards of economic theory, a powerful congruence of interests may emerge. Market relations are extended to the medical care system in a way that relegates providers to a secondary role. Either the state or business tells hospitals and physicians how to be organized, how to treat patients, and how much to charge.[30] Thus, the power of business may be the central theme that weaves politics, power, and policy into a whole tapestry.

3

Business and the Pushcart Vendors

IN JULY 1969, Richard Nixon's secretary of health, education and welfare, Robert H. Finch, declared, "We will ask and challenge American business to involve itself in the health care industry, including the creation of new and competitive forms of organization to deliver comprehensive health services on a large scale."[1]

The Background of Business Participation

How did business get so involved in the politics of health care in the past decade, and why is 1969 an important year with which to begin this discussion? It is an important date because 1969 marks the beginning of a decline in corporate profits accompanied by a national involvement of both business and government in reorganizing and rationalizing health care. A leading business journal declared in 1970, "Our present system of medical care is not a system at all. The majority of physicians constitute an *army of pushcart vendors in an age of supermarkets.*"[2] Both politics and economics propelled business into its widespread and active role in changing health policy and bringing the independent physicians and institutions into the American health care supermarket.

This chapter describes both the American economy of the 1960s and 1970s and the role business played in public policy debates as a result of world economic conditions, relates how American business entered into the health policy debate of the 1970s and 1980s, and documents the way in which business interest was expressed in both the health policy and business journals of the latter two decades.

Of course, the involvement of American business in reorganizing the medical care industry did *not* begin in 1969. American corporations have been actively involved in health care throughout this century; for example, major foundations, such as the Rockefeller and Carnegie, have intervened in issues of worker injury, public health sanitation, and medical education. The active intervention of businessmen, like Henry J. Kaiser, who began building hospitals and clinics for his workers in the 1920s, also worked directly for reforms.[3] One of the most significant attempts of corporations and foundations to restructure medical care was the research of the Committee on the Costs of Medical Care, whose findings were released in 1933.[4] This report called for a number of reforms that seem commonplace now, such as group practice of physicians, voluntary group insurance, geographic coordination of services, and the general rationalization of medical care.

In addition to the current wave of intervention, there have been three waves of corporate intervention in the medical sector in the past hundred years, roughly corresponding to predepression phases of long-term economic cycles sometimes called Kuznets cycles (1888–1893, 1904–1910, and 1925–1933).[5] These boom periods were characterized by rising interest rates and prices. The end of these periods also marked the beginning of a general profit squeeze on business during which time major segments of business sought ways to reduce their costs.

At first glance the strong associations between economic conditions and political activism seem causally related. For example, corporate interest in issues of public health and sanitation in the early 1900s was preceded by intense labor unrest in the late 1800s, the development of a germ theory, and links between poor sanitation and disease. The interventions of the Rockefeller Foundation and the release of the Flexner Report occurred between 1905 and 1914, corresponding to the second Kuznets economic cycle, and the Committee on Cost of Medical Care carried out its work between 1926 and 1933, approximately the period of the third cycle.[6] As Salmon has noted, these business interventions appeared to be designed to modify and transform the medical care system to better accommodate a developing capitalist economy. Whether these interventions were caused by the economic cycles has not yet been proven.[7]

Other business interventions during and after World War II related to the development of Blue Cross and Blue Shield insurance in the late 1930s and the use of fringe benefits as a bargaining tool by labor in the late 1940s and 1950s. According to current President of Blue Cross Bernard Tresnowski, business was not actively involved in developing the Blue Cross idea; hospitals and doctors pushed the concept. However, once the discussion began, business became interested in whether the principles of insurance could be applied to health care and supported the development of a nonprofit "health service plan" model that later was called Blue Cross.[8]

The introduction of health benefits into the collective bargaining process and the expanded benefits labor won in the 1950s provided part of the context in which management began to be concerned with health care costs in the late 1960s. When Medicare and Medicaid were being discussed and enacted in the mid-1960s, according to Walter McNerney, former president of Blue Cross, business was more reactive than proactive. "Management made its point of view known mainly to emphasize its concerns about minimizing costs and keeping private sector control over insurance and delivery aspects of the programs."[9] But not until the economy tumbled in the late 1960s and the costs of Medicare and Medicaid skyrocketed, prompting cost shifts to the private sector, did business begin its latest and most aggressive intervention in the health care sector.

Business and the Economy: 1969–1980

The American economy of the late 1960s and early 1970s was marked by the lowest level of corporate profits in the share of national income since World War II.[10] "Few events discipline the corporate mind as fast as a drop in earnings."[11] Pretax rates of return for nonfinancial corporations dropped from a high of 13.7 percent in 1965 (the highest rate since 1948–1949) to 8.1 percent in 1970. Aftertax rates of return followed a similar pattern, declining from a high of 10.3 percent in 1965 to 5.9 percent in 1970.[12] A third plunge in corporate profits occurred in the early 1980s, when, according to a study by Data Resources, the inflation-adjusted profit rate in 1982 had reached its lowest level since the early 1970s.[13]

Some causes of this decline in profits included the debt financing of the Viet Nam War and the costs of the Great Society, including Medicare and Medicaid that had passed in 1966 but had already begun to show cost increases in 1968. "The trade surplus had begun to decline in 1966, and by 1971 it turned negative for the first time in the twentieth century."[14] What many economists had predicted would be a boom decade in the 1970s started out with a recession in 1969 and 1970, increasing inflation, shortages of critical raw materials, and an erosion of the financial markets in the early 1970s.

President Nixon's unprecedented wage and price controls in the early 1970s did not stem inflation, and the economic prognosticators, although accurately predicting vigorous economic growth and rising real incomes, did not foresee some obstacles to a stable and continued growth. How-ever, in the early 1970s economists failed to predict either a worldwide shortage of raw materials such as metals, timber, and oil or the power the oil cartel would hold, both economically and politically, in the world mar-kets. While they forecast continuing inflation, they thought it would peak at about 4 percent a year. They missed the inflationary explosion of 1973–1974 that drove price increases in the United States to 12 percent and over 100 percent in some developing countries.[15]

The economists expected a certain degree of increased intervention by government in regulating health, safety, and the environment, but not the costs that regulation would impose on industry for enforcing compli-ance (e.g., the passage of the Coal Mine Safety Act of 1969, the Occupa-tional Health and Safety Act of 1970, the Rehabilitation Act of 1973, and the Toxic Substances Control Act of 1976).[16] They forecast rising de-mands for investment and capital, but not the breakdown of the system of financial markets at the moment when business most needed access to capital. As *Business Week* noted in 1974, "Perhaps the most important single development of the first half of the Seventies has been the creation of a truly international, worldwide economy that has a life of its own."[17]

Economists, as well as politicians, had also failed to foresee the inevi-table political changes when independent governments in Third World countries that controlled key resources began to use those resources as bargaining chips in world politics. American banks were only too happy to loan money on the worldwide market, although brokerage houses col-lapsed and the stock market began to weaken under the weight of the debilitating inflation. By mid-1974, accompanied by a general decline in public confidence, American business faced a major challenge to rebuild the country's investment machinery and increase labor's productivity. The alternatives were grim: continuing trends of declining profits and an increasing political and economic burden of government regulation. Business was also confronted with the cost of health benefits that had been richly negotiated in previous decades. Despite the weakness of American labor in the 1970s, the benefit plans were already in place, and business had only recently become aware of the way in which their pre-miums were increasing.

Business, Health Care Costs, and the Pushcart Vendors

By the early 1970s, business had been challenged by economic condi-tions to pay attention to a drain on profit that affected the health of both their workers and their companies: the American health care industry.

When a few chief executive officers from large business firms such as New York Telephone and Duquesne Light Company were interviewed in 1970, they commented, "Business has a sizable stake in health insurance, if only because it is a costly fringe benefit that companies pay to millions of workers."[18] Americans are now inured to hearing about 20 percent annual increases in health insurance premiums, but in the late 1960s, business costs per employee for health insurance increased 27 percent in one year, prompting some larger corporations to take notice. New York Telephone paid about half the total health care bill for employees in 1967; by 1970 it was covering the entire package. "We are very concerned about the inflation in medical costs," understated one spokesman.[19]

Employers continued to pay more of the total cost of health insurance for their employees, and the costs of medical care continued to increase throughout the 1970s. From 1967 to 1978, according to a study by the U.S. Chamber of Commerce, the average benefits paid by employers for health related items, including social security taxes, increased from $10.90 to $38.99 per week per employee; all employee benefits as a portion of total payroll increased from 29.1 percent to 41.2 percent in the same period. In 1976, the average company spent 5.1 percent of its payroll on health benefits; by 1978 it was up to 5.8 percent; by 1984, it averaged 8 percent nationwide, and by 1987 it had reached 9.7 percent. Private employers were financing nearly one of every five dollars spent on health care in America by 1984.[20]

An index of corporate profitability considered by many economists to be a better measure of corporate strength than aftertax income is the rate of return earned by nonfinancial businesses on the value of their plants, machinery, and equipment. A survey of changes in corporate profitability since 1948 shows that corporations earned an 8 percent rate of return in 1948, 5 percent in 1960, 8 percent again in 1965, and then there has been a steady plunge downward, reaching 3.8 percent in 1970, 2.1 percent in 1974, and 2 percent in 1982. A rebound that began in 1983 had only reached 4.2 percent by the end of 1986.[21] If there is a connection between economic recessions, corporate profitability, and interventions in health care, then the major corporations should have begun to become concerned in the 1970s, with a peak of activity occurring in the mid-1970s and again in the early and mid-1980s. That is exactly what happened.

Not every CEO of a major corporation realized the connection between medical care increases and eroding corporate profits, and even those who recognized the issue did not always place it high on an agenda for action. However, that a significant "dominant segment" of the corporate elite did recognize the dilemma is revealed by several indicators: the number of articles in the business press devoted to the health care crisis; the release of the influential Committee for Economic Development's report on health care costs in 1973 and reports by the Conference Board and Business Council; and the formation of various task forces and associations to deal with health care issues, such as the Washington Business Group on Health by the Business Roundtable in 1974.[22]

As the health of the general economy declined in the early 1970s, the medical care industry itself boomed. In the early 1970s, business had no intention of destroying that growth; it simply wanted to rationalize and direct it more efficiently. Within a few days of each other, in January 1970, both *Fortune* magazine and *Business Week* carried cover stories on the American medical industry and the need for business to become involved in reorganizing it more efficiently. *Fortune* declared its agenda in a series of articles, all emphasizing cost containment, efficiency, and better management: "It's Time to Operate," "Hospitals Need Management Even More Than Money," "Better Care at Less Cost without Miracles," "Change Begins in the Doctor's Office," and "The Medical Industrial Complex."

The opening editorial of the *Fortune* article was an explicit volley from the business community to the medical care industry and government. "American medicine . . . stands now on the brink of chaos. Much of U.S. medical care . . . is inferior in quality, wastefully dispensed, and inequitably financed." The article continued, "The time has come for radical change. . . . The management of medical care has become too important to leave to doctors, who are, after all, not managers to begin with."[23]

The remainder of the articles formed a searing indictment of the way medicine was practiced, a critique that was a clear example of the ideology of corporate rationalization. Some elements that link "corporate rationalizers" are "an understanding of the increasing social and complex division of labor within the medical care system; an appreciation of the importance of the hospital as a site for organizing complex technology; and a commitment to cost control which may involve breaking the professional monopoly of physicians over the production and distribution of medical care services."[24] In the 1970s, the corporatization of American health care had just begun, and the drive to stabilize the health care industry was being promoted more by the businesses that purchased health care than by those that produced it.

Paul Ellwood, a physician who had formed InterStudy in the 1970s, a think tank for the research and development of health maintenance organizations (HMOs), and who was the main architect of President Nixon's HMO strategy, saw no problem with corporations running health care. Others viewed organized medicine and the insurance industry with suspicion. "The biggest obstacle to a more rational medical system . . . is organized medicine," Faltermayer declared in the *Fortune* article. Then he added, "Private insurers need to exert greater control over medical costs."[25] Another article in *Fortune* stated, "Basic structural reforms are needed to give the system permanent stability . . . in business . . . the profit motive spurs efficiency, and some believe it could do the same for hospitals."[26] The themes were clear. Growth in the medical care industry is acceptable to the rest of American business and even desirable, if it proceeds in an efficient manner, contributes to the health of workers, and does not drain other sectors of American business.

The Health Care Crisis and the American Press

One way of tracking a social issue and trying to decide who has the most power over its definition and solutions is to scan the media for references to the problem. Not only can the frequency of articles on a given subject indicate the salience of that subject for public policy, but the type of press in which the issue is discussed can also indicate the sectors of society most concerned with the issue. As Arnold Rose has noted, "There can be little doubt that those who own and manage most of the newspapers of the United States are more pro-business than they are supportive of any other segment of the population."[27]

In the case of health care, starting in the 1970s, most major business magazines, as well as *The New York Times* and *The Wall Street Journal*, began to carry lead articles on the subject of health care costs. In the 1970s and 1980s the number of articles in the business press addressing business's role in health care cost containment steadily increased. In a computerized search of articles in *Forbes, Fortune,* and *Business Week,* between 1972 and 1988, using the key words "health," "medical," or "medicine," and "cost," "control," or "containment," 308 articles were located, with the largest number of articles in any two-year period appearing in 1984–1985 (see Table 3.1).[28]

In a computerized search of articles in *The New York Times* between 1980 (the first year a computerized search was available) and mid-1988, using "business" or "corporate" and "health care costs" as key words, 131 articles were located linking business efforts with health care cost containment (see Table 3.2). The number of articles on this topic steadily increased through 1987, and, although I ended the search in mid-1988, 17 articles were located in the first six months of 1988, demonstrating no particular decrease in interest in the topic throughout the decade.

Of note is the fact that *The New York Times* is a newspaper whose "broad readership tends to favor general corporate coverage over specific

TABLE 3.1   *Frequency of Articles Relating Business to Health Care Cost Containment in* Fortune, Forbes, *and* Business Week, *1972–1988*

YEARS	NUMBER OF ARTICLES APPEARING IN ANY OF THESE MAGAZINES IN A TWO-YEAR PERIOD
1970–1971	*database not available*
1972–1973[a]	7
1974–1975	17
1976–1977	24
1978–1979	43
1980–1981	25
1982–1983	52
1984–1985	82
1986–1988[b]	58

Source: Computerized database compiled by author searching issues of *Fortune, Forbes,* and *Business Week* between January 1971 and June 1988.
[a]The *Business Week* database does not begin until November 1972.
[b]The 1988 count includes only January through June.

TABLE 3.2   *Frequency of Articles in the* New York Times *Mentioning Business and Health Care Cost Containment, 1980–1988*

YEAR	GENERAL ARTICLES	BUSINESS & HEALTH ARTICLES	TOTAL
1980	2	—	2
1981	3	—	3
1982	8	—	8
1983	7	—	7
1984	19	—	19
1985	16	9[a]	25
1986	13	8	21
1987	11	18	29
1988[b]	5	12	17
Total	84	47	131

Source: Computerized search of articles by author mentioning either business or corporations and health care/cost containment in the *New York Times* between 1980 and 1988.
[a]A special column entitled "Business and Health" was instituted by the *New York Times* in 1985.
[b]Articles for 1988 include January through June only.

company affairs. Quotation or citation in *The New York Times* can serve as a suitable sign of access to the media." A study done by Michael Useem showed that the "inner circle seeks out, and is accorded, greater access than other business leaders to those broad publics served by the print media."[29] Therefore, it seems reasonable to expect that if the issue of health care cost containment was of importance to business and if business wanted to get that word out to the rest of the corporate and policy community, *The New York Times* would be likely to carry an increasing number of stories on the subject. The subject of health care cost containment became so important to the business readership of the *Times* by 1985 that a special column called "Business and Health" was added to the Business Section of the *Times,* and between 1985 and mid-1988 forty-seven columns were run on that topic alone.

A "health care crisis" had been announced by the business press in *Business Week*'s January 1970 "Special Report" entitled "The $60 Billion Crisis Over Medical Care." The theme of "crisis" occurred over and over again during the 1970s, mainly in the business press, although increasingly mentioned in health journals during the latter half of the decade. A scan of the substance of these articles reveals little mention of any sources of "crisis" other than inefficiency or even the implications of inefficiency in the medical care sector for other sectors of American business. Indeed, declaring a crisis seemed a necessary prelude to the inevitable next step, offering solutions.

Certain solutions emerged in the press in the 1970s, calling for "cost control" to ameliorate the crisis. The solutions that business proposed in the early 1970s were diverse. *Business Week* editors proposed a national health insurance plan and/or promoted more efficient group practices such as the Kaiser Permanente Health Maintenance Organization. The article quoted several academic economists who all proposed management or efficiency solutions as the way to solve the crisis. Of the one hundred firms questioned by *Business Week,* most had an "open mind" about national health insurance (NHI), but only a few were willing to support it unequivocally. One executive said, "If what I've been reading about health care in this country today is true, then standing up against a national health plan would be like arguing against God and motherhood. . . . My snap opinion is that a national plan would involve constantly escalating costs. But more important, a national plan would take away an item worth up to a cent an hour that you can now stack on the bargaining table."[30]

The 1970 *Business Week* article provided the first comprehensive treatment ever given national health insurance in a national business magazine. The four major bills being proposed by the Nixon administration and Congress were reviewed, and the political advantages and disadvantages pointed out. "Reforming the medical system is an idea whose time has come," one NHI supporter was quoted as saying. Well, not quite. The Nixon health care reformers saw their liaison with American business much the way the Reagan administration supporters did a decade later. There was a crisis; it needed a solution; and American business could provide that support. The article concluded: "Backers of a national plan see this as a good chance to get in an opening wedge."[31] Even though the right wing defeated the moderates on national health insurance in the 1970s and the Business Roundtable and the Washington Business Group on Health expressed their strong reservations about it, the very real economic constraints on the profitability of American business gave liberal health policy advocates an opening in the window (or the door) of opportunity in 1970.

The HMO Strategy

Between 1969 and 1974, there was a series of articles in both government and business periodicals about HMOs and their potential for solving the health care crisis. Hardly a month passed without an article in the *Harvard Business Review, Fortune, Business Week, The Wall Street Journal,* or *The New York Times* about the way HMOs could help rationalize the American medical care system. It was all a way of educating American business and the consumer public about the problem and getting solutions in place that would not jeopardize the private financing and delivery of American medical care.[32] Nixon's 1971 State of the Union speech mentioned health maintenance organizations as the cornerstone of restructuring the American health care system. Again, organized medicine was spotlighted as the chief obstacle to these changes, and they remained openly opposed to the concept.

In 1973, several important events occurred: The HMO Act of 1973 was passed, giving federal support and subsidy to the development of HMOs all over the country. Paul Ellwood urged corporations to get involved and offer HMO options to their employees, and many corporations did. Evidence of corporate interest in this solution to the health care crisis can be found in the 1973 Committee for Economic Development policy paper, "Building a National Health Care System." It was very much the product of big business, with its comprehensive solutions of rationality, better management, more efficiency, without challenging the private control over the delivery of health care services in the United States. There was, however, a glint of recognition that business might have to do more than support HMOs or national health insurance in order to reform the medical care system.[33]

The physicians and drug manufacturers who participated in the CED policy discussion wrote dissenting reports arguing against prepayment for health care, government interference, and, indeed, any interference with the status quo. But three businessmen, representing large banking and manufacturing firms, also dissented. They agreed that a national health care system was important, but they pleaded for both the creation of a "true market" with patient choice among competing modes of delivery and a "major role for private capital and management paralleling the rest of the nation's industrial system." They concluded, "Our health-care industry is the only major industry that has not had to submit to the discipline either of the marketplace or of public regulation."[34]

Although American business was in no way committed to the task of disciplining the medical care sector alone in 1973, a warning note had been sounded. No sector of industry could continue to grow as fast as medical care if it was to be at the substantial expense of the rest of the industrial community, and no individual entrepreneurs, such as physicians, could continue to control the rate of growth in medical services without accountability to the purchasers. The pushcart vendors were about to be brought inside the supermarket but not without a fight.

The recession of 1974 intervened to provide physicians with a short period of relief from the corporate takeover of medicine, while business attempted to define its strategy. However, medical care costs neither substantially declined during the recession, nor did HMOs take off in the way their promoters had envisioned. A *Business Week* article declared in January 1975, "Still Waiting for HMOs," and *The Wall Street Journal* wrote the next month, "HMOs Falter."

Business and the Regulatory Approach

In 1974, government, attempting to rationalize the medical care industry through regulation, passed a national health planning act, Public Law 93-641, that created a network of over two hundred planning agencies all over the country. Planning and certificate of need regulation of health facility expansion were to be the cornerstones of the new rational system. Educated and aggressive consumer majorities on the planning boards were brought in to balance the power of organized medicine. Business was ambivalent about the role of planning and regulation, an ambivalence that would continue through the 1970s and into the 1980s, reflecting the divisions between large and small business, businesses that provided medical care services or manufactured medical devices, and businesses that mainly purchased health insurance for their employees.

The 1970 *Fortune* article had warned about the stake of American industry in the "medical industrial complex." Almost every major corporation in the country had a subsidiary with some stake in the growth of the medical sector, and the government had made that growth both possible and inevitable. Therefore, a too aggressive restriction on the growth of the medical care sector could and would affect all types of business in the United States. These divisions within business help explain its ambivalence toward regulatory solutions in general and health care specifically.

Until 1976, the complex relationship between business and the state over issues of the medical care crisis and its potential solutions had surfaced mainly in the business or government press. With the movement toward liberal politics demonstrated by the election of President Jimmy Carter and other Democratic liberals in 1976, the climate toward business changed unexpectedly, and health professionals began to recognize the importance and contributions of American business to health policy change. *Perspective*, the journal published by Blue Cross, ran articles in its 1977 winter and spring issues about the strategies of the U.S. Chamber of Commerce, the Washington Business Group on Health, and major corporations regarding health care cost containment. The community of health professionals had begun to wake up to the fact that increases in health care premiums hurt business profitability and that business had a stake in changing the system.

Carter's administration also opened up a new relationship between the executive branch and big business that had been somewhat dormant or even outright antagonistic during the Nixon and Ford administrations, according to executives such as Irving Shapiro of du Pont Corporation.[35] The Council on Wage and Price Stability released a major policy statement in 1976, calling attention to the need for business to become active in controlling health care costs:

> There is no evidence that health care providers, left to their own devices, would do anything other than to behave in a manner which will continue to fuel an inflationary bias already deeply imbedded in the structure of the system. . . . We are convinced that an alternative to federal control of the health care system is available.
>
> If promptly seized . . . that alternative is a concerted and united effort on the part of industry and labor to control costs.[36]

Business had begun to emerge from more than a decade of recession and retreat into a newly energized public policy role, partially stimulated by a generally increased government regulation of industry. Medical care began to attain more importance on the agenda of businesses outside the dominant segment of corporate elites, as costs continued to increase and no proposed solutions seemed to be working. Under Carter, talk about HMOs was revived, and government regulation of medical care costs became more than an idle threat. Once again physicians came under fire. *The Wall Street Journal* ran an editorial in January 1977, "Health Care: Ripe for Regulation," followed by a *Forbes* article in October 1977, "Physician Heal Thyself . . . Or Else!" In 1977 and 1978, corporations even began to start their own HMOs, getting widespread press attention for their efforts.[37]

Through the efforts of Professor John T. Dunlop of Harvard University, a former U.S. secretary of labor, an informal group of prominent labor and business leaders met and published in 1978 a position paper on health care costs. This was one of the first position papers put together by leaders of both labor and management on the issue of health care cost containment. Although labor still supported national health insurance as a solution, it did not stop the leadership from agreeing on the need for concerted action by all parties.

At the state and local level, companies had begun to develop internal strategies about cutting costs of health care premiums. Many of those early strategies involved shifting costs from management to labor, although requiring employees to pay higher deductibles did not take off until 1983. The shift in deductibles previously paid by management to more recent payment by labor has been rapid: In 1979, 14 percent of large corporations required employees to pay a deductible for medical expenses; in 1982, it was 17 percent; in 1983, it had grown to 32 percent, and by 1984, 52 percent.[38]

Neither attempts by the Carter administration to slow down health care costs by various marginal regulatory controls nor the loudly advertized "voluntary effort" by hospitals to keep their own costs down produced substantial cost containment, however. By the end of the 1970s, health care costs were still increasing, and business had not yet found a satisfactory mechanism by which to control them. Companies also began to work together more effectively, forming business coalitions, alliances, roundtables, and informal networks to talk about medical care costs and possible solutions. It is the challenge to business interests that induces business to organize itself politically. Once the challenge has been dealt with, business organizations persist. As Graham Wilson explains, "It is the past, not the current character of the challenge to business which explains the degree of its current organization."[39]

4

Institutional Mechanisms for Change

Our biggest job is to change the way business behaves. . . . If you want to change institutions, then you have to look at how institutions change. The history of American business involvement is that they create an "institutional mechanism" to guide their change, after they have identified something as worthy of change.

— Willis Goldbeck, interview

As I HAVE SHOWN in Chapter 3, economic and political forces propelled business into active political participation in health policy in the 1970s and 1980s. The task of business in the mid-1970s was to develop the mechanisms for change that it would implement in the 1980s. These institutional mechanisms are the keys to an effective public policy strategy for business, according to business representatives such as Willis Goldbeck of the Washington Business Group on Health,[1] Irving Shapiro of du Pont and the Business Roundtable, and academics as diverse as John T. Dunlop of Harvard University and G. William Domhoff of the University of California.[2]

Although many national organizations have addressed health care issues in the last two decades, this chapter will focus on several national organizational mechanisms for change supported or created by business representatives to implement their health policy agenda between 1974 and 1988: (1) Chamber of Commerce of the U.S. and its health care task force; (2) National Business Roundtable and its health care task force; (3) Washington Business Group on Health; (4) Dunlop Group of Six; and (5) local or regional business and health coalitions. How do these organizations work? How did they come to be involved with health policy issues? And what policy positions did they support? These questions illuminate the way in which business influences the policy process.

National Institutional Mechanisms:
Chamber of Commerce of the United States

Of the three national business organizations that showed an interest in health care politics in the late 1970s and early 1980s, the Chamber of Commerce of the U.S. was both the oldest and the most favored by the Reagan administration. Founded in 1912 with the help of corporate liberals as well as the National Association of Manufacturers (NAM—itself founded in 1894), the Chamber became an association of associations encompassing all sizes and types of U.S. business, including manufacturing, service, retail, construction, finance, transportation, and agriculture. Although the average size of member firms was smaller than NAM (87 percent of the member firms had fewer than fifty employees) and its ideology promoted its dedication to small business, the Chamber was and still is, at least to some degree, controlled by big business through its policy committees. Of sixty-four directors in 1981, twenty-four (38 percent) were from Fortune 500 companies.[3]

By the 1980s the Chamber of Commerce of the U.S. was growing rapidly. Its membership had quadrupled between 1976 and 1982, with the biggest gain coming between April 1981 and June 1982. Companies with less than ten employees accounted for 70 percent of the increase in membership during the years of the Reagan administration. The Chamber had used its connections with the White House to fuel its membership drive. The Chamber mobilized its 2,700 state and local chambers, 1,400 member trade associations, and 165,000 member companies in 1981 to support the president's tax and budget proposals. As Reagan's Special Liaison with Business Wayne Valis, said, "Different groups may match the Chamber in a specific area, but with their media programs, Hill contacts, and grass-roots organization, nothing can match them in overall effectiveness. They're simply in a class by themselves."[4]

Along with an increase in membership came an increase in organizational activity and staffing. By 1982 the Chamber had thirty internal committees, fourteen hundred staff members in Washington, and another six hundred staff members in the field. With the diversity of interests and members and the rapidly increasing number of employees, it is not surprising that many members felt that the Chamber staff controlled policy decisions. Another factor limiting the Chamber's effectiveness was that providers were often chairs of the health committees, causing some conflict among business members over policy choices. Thirty policy committees met only infrequently, and policy had to be approved by these committees and then sent to the board for final ratification before the Chamber could take any position.[5]

At the beginning of 1981, the Chamber declared publicly that it would support the president's health proposals down the line. The line was short, however. Once a tax on employer paid health premium contributions was proposed, the Chamber drew back. And when health care for the unemployed was discussed, the Chamber would not even admit the existence of an unemployment problem.[6]

The Chamber's effectiveness in influencing health policy began to be questioned when David Winston began his work as special consultant to the White House in mid-1982. Winston was given the responsibility of pulling together White House health policy and bringing the business community along. He commented, "We had no widespread support from the business community and we began asking why. The staff were so in charge of the organization, that the Chamber had even come out explicitly for hospital rate setting. Oh, they had a euphemism for it, 'state efforts to control health care costs,' but the staff translated that into support for rate setting."[7]

So Winston and a few White House people decided to have a "little talk" with the Chamber. "We had a very interesting and constructive meeting with the President of the Chamber, Richard Lesher. We said, 'We're for free enterprise and competition and we don't understand why you're not.' And he was shocked. 'What do you mean?' he said. And we replied, 'Why do you want to have the health business, which is the third largest business in the country, put under regulatory controls when you have been traditionally opposed to regulatory controls?" Winston recalled that Lesher was unaware of a position paper that the Chamber health care committee was about to vote on the very next week, and, encouraged by Winston and the White House, Lesher exerted his authority instantly. The Chamber voted against the staff position and cleaned up its language about "state efforts" at the very next meeting.

About the same time, Winston decided that Lesher needed to know about the dominance of commercial insurers and their support for health care regulation in the Chamber's health policy committees. Winston and several others invited Lesher to Project HOPE (one of the White House's favorite think tanks) in Millwood, Virginia, for another little talk. "It had become clear to us," said Winston, "that the committees were stacked in favor of insurers. We had a lot of work to do to be sure that the committee became balanced." Winston and the administration encouraged Lesher to reassert control, of both his own staff and his policy committees. The commercial insurers were powerful when left alone on committees but not nearly so powerful when confronted with a full roster of the other interests such as business representatives, hospitals, physicians, and Blue Cross.[8]

Probably the biggest contribution that the Chamber made to the participation and involvement of business in health policy issues in the

1980s was to support the growing business coalition movement through its Clearinghouse on Business Coalitions for Health Action. Although it helped create awareness among chambers around the country, not until 1982 did local chambers really begin to participate seriously in local health coalitions. In 1982 the Clearinghouse reported only 25 coalitions, but 150 coalitions responded to Chamber surveys by April 1984. The Clearinghouse directory stated, "The purpose of the Clearinghouse is to help promote the growth and development of coalitions through the preparation, collection and dissemination of business and health information and of data specifically for or about coalitions."[9]

In 1984 the Chamber somewhat changed the coalition membership categories and character; the alterations reflected the Chamber's growing awareness of the different interests and variations in policy orientation of health-related and non-health-related business, as well as the changing role of the state from regulator to purchaser. For the first time the business category was divided into categories of firms in the "health care business" (e.g., pharmaceutical companies, hospital suppliers, etc.) and those that were not (e.g., auto manufacturers, petroleum industries, etc.). The health category was divided into physician, hospital, and insurance/health plan members, and government was given two divisions—one for regulators (i.e., health systems agencies) and one for purchasers (i.e., city government, school boards, etc.). These changes reflected a similar debate in local coalitions all over the country about who represented whom for what purpose.

Despite the efforts of Winston and others at the national level, health care providers maintained their domination over the Chamber's health policy committees at the local and state level. The ability of local chambers to take positions that would challenge the power of community health care providers who were also Chamber members varied greatly from community to community. In California in 1982, the state Chamber of Commerce was unusually active in the policy process, primarily because the Chamber staff member had been a state legislative staff member and was able to pull together skillfully the fragmented Chamber members. In Massachusetts, the state Chamber was not significantly involved with the 1982 legislation, although shortly afterward they formed a new health advisory group in competition with the Massachusetts Business Roundtable.

Because of its blanket endorsement of most Reagan policies, its domination by small business and provider interests, and its slow-moving policy process, the national Chamber was unable to respond quickly to new twists and turns in legislation and was not regarded by congressional decision makers as wielding the same level of power as some other organizations more openly identified with big business, such as the Roundtable or WBGH. By the mid-1980s, the Chamber of Commerce of the U.S. had turned over its coalition directory activities to the American Hospital Association, and the activities of its health care task force slowed down considerably.

The Business Roundtable

The Business Roundtable, founded in 1972 to give big business more clout in Washington, was quite different from the Chamber of Commerce in that, unlike the Chamber or NAM, its own members ran the organization. Each task force was chaired by a CEO, and all task force work was done by staff within the company of that CEO. Although the original Roundtable was intended to be a small group of influential business leaders, within ten years it had grown to more than two hundred members with sixteen task forces. Membership was invited, and the list was not made public. However, an unofficial list suggested that of the fifty largest corporations in the United States in 1975, only thirteen did *not* belong to the Roundtable: five oil companies, plus Lockheed, W. R. Grace, Beatrice Foods, I. T. and T., Eastman Kodak, Borden, and Amerada Hess Corporation. Unofficial estimates stated that the Business Roundtable membership included 131 of the top 500 corporations on the Fortune 500 list.[10]

From the very beginning, the Roundtable was designed to lobby more actively than the Business Council, another powerful national business organization. Although it never registered as an organizational lobbyist, everyone agreed that the Roundtable would aggressively work on issues of national importance, whether it be called lobbying or not. The Roundtable members themselves were determined to do the background work on issues and to present their viewpoints themselves to legislators and presidential advisers. During the Carter administration, position papers were prepared for the president on various issues, and the leaders of the Roundtable were often consulted by the White House.[11]

The policy issues discussed and supported by the Roundtable had to meet two criteria: the problem had to have an impact on both member companies and the economic well-being of the country. Medicare and health care costs met both criteria. Although the Roundtable later expanded its health policy menu in the 1980s to include the uninsured and the taxation of benefits, the issues that the Roundtable's Health Care Task Force addressed in the mid-1970s were much more narrowly related to the interests of the drug industry and its major spokesman, the Eli Lilly Company, whose representative also chaired the Roundtable's task force. One Roundtable business member whose firm was also a member of WBGH said, "The agenda of the Health Care Task Force of the BR changed considerably when Eli Lilly company took it over. We were told, informally by Capitol Hill staff members, that the effectiveness of the BR was diluted when Lilly people would appear on the Hill one week to lobby for drug bills and come back the next week claiming to represent the Roundtable."[12]

When the Roundtable's Health Care Task Force was formed, Walter Wriston of Citibank provided the leadership. When Wriston stepped down and Eli Lilly stepped in, the purity of purchaser power was diluted. Throughout the remainder of the 1970s and 1980s, with drug companies and insurance companies providing task force leadership, many observers noted that the conflicts of interest between individual company agendas and national policy issues resulted in fewer and less strongly stated positions by the Roundtable on critical issues of health policy.[13]

On health issues the Roundtable delegated issues to the vice presidents in charge of employee benefits, who also often worked with the WBGH. David Winston commented, "Many CEOs have no idea in the world what is being said by the WBGH on their behalf, or probably the Roundtable for that matter. But they would be more likely to know what is going on at the Roundtable because they themselves attend meetings." In 1984 the WBGH policy director noted, "There's about 60 percent overlap between the Roundtable and WBGH, and we do tend to have benefit managers rather than CEOs attend our meetings. Some of the CEOs wouldn't like what we're saying on behalf of business if they knew it, but at some level it suits their needs for us to be saying what we do. Sometimes it's to their advantage to complain publicly but allow things to continue as usual within the organization."[14]

During the policy formation process of the 1980s, the Roundtable was involved in the health policy debate in a number of other ways: the Health Care Task Force of the Roundtable continued to meet; regional seminars on health policy were organized by task force CEOs around the country; Walter Wriston of the Business Roundtable agreed to participate in the Dunlop Group of Six (see discussion later in this chapter); and the Roundtable issued policy papers. "An Appropriate Role for Corporations in Health Care Cost Management" released in February 1982 outlined the Roundtable's health care strategy.[15]

The Roundtable program as outlined in the policy paper was not particularly strong. It encouraged CEOs to exercise "leadership in addressing local issues in the health care delivery system within the parameters of law and regulation. Local action can be instrumental in slowing the rise in costs, but it is not appropriate to tinker unduly with systems that are among the best in the world." Three strategies were proposed to achieve Roundtable goals: (1) local action—leadership roles in demonstration projects; (2) cost management—supporting intracompany cost-containment efforts, increased involvement in local coalitions, and encouraging employer participation in hospital management through better trustee training programs; and (3) research—how to contain costs and keep good quality health care. The paper emphasized business leadership in coalitions, planning agencies, and hospital boards. While acknowledging the reality that solutions could be effective only if all interested groups cooperated, the report also stated, "Employer-only coalitions should be encouraged." This support of local coalitions might not be a surprising suggestion, except that only a year before this paper was produced, a special vote had to be taken at the Roundtable Board to allow Walter Wriston, the Health Care Committee's chairman, and his representative on the Dunlop Group, Chris York, to lend Roundtable support for developing coalitions including business on the local level. Roundtable policy had previously been directed only to national issues.[16]

In 1984, John Creedon of Metropolitan Life merged the work of the Business Roundtable health care task force with the welfare and retirement task force into one group called "Health, Welfare and Retirement Income." This reorganization occurred because these issues paralleled the government's major entitlement programs such as social security, Medicare, and Medicaid, which faced declining public revenues and an aging population. The newly reorganized task force tackled two issues in 1985 and 1986: the taxation of employer-paid health benefits and the mandated extension of employee benefits after job termination through the Consolidated Omnibus Reconciliation Act of 1985 (COBRA). The Business Roundtable decided to oppose both proposals. The taxation of benefits never passed the Congress, but the "mandated" extension of benefits after the termination of employment passed, partially by being embedded in the budget process. According to task force staff, "That was the first piece of legislation that got through us in the reconciliation process that was of interest to business and this task force." A Roundtable staff member commented that the best way to avoid such losses was to keep issues off the agenda completely, although he admitted that was not always easy.

The Washington Business Group on Health

Ultimately, the Roundtable was most comfortable leaving the details of health policy to the organization it had created in the mid-1970s to do its dirty work, the Washington Business Group on Health. Health care had been one of the Roundtable's issues of concern at its formation. The first chairman of the health care task force in 1973 was Henry Ford II. But Ford did not want to staff the health care task force with his own people, so he delegated Rod Marklee and Bill White of U.S. Steel to put together a staff. According to Willis Goldbeck, who was eventually chosen to staff the health care group, the selection process was typical of the informal relationships and processes among the business elite:

> I took a totally different approach from the others. . . . They all wanted to teach these Washington people how to lobby health. I said, "What you want is someone who will preclude the necessity for you having to be taught how to lobby on health. The objective is for big business to become a credible participant in national health policy."
>
> Ford Motor Company gave me a check for $5,000 and gave me thirty days to start an organization and pay them back or disappear. I said, "Fine, but this is what I want: (1) I want it to be my existing corporation; ·(2) I want it to be independent of the Roundtable but have all the Roundtable participating in it; (3) I want 100 percent authority over it other than reporting to Marklee personally; and (4) I want to be able to include non Roundtable companies in the organization." They said, "If you can do that in thirty days, it's probably the right thing to do," and they snickered and walked away. Thirty days later I gave him his check back, and we've been in business ever since.

The Washington Business Group on Health very quickly moved out in front of the Roundtable on health issues in a number of ways. In spite of the fact that Goldbeck was not in business and felt uncomfortable with businessmen, he became the maverick leader of what he called an "institutional mechanism for social change." Goldbeck's ideas and role are emphasized here for a number of reasons. For the first few years, Goldbeck was the most visible representative of the WBGH. Except for secretarial support, he was the only staff member, and his ideas were often considerably more progressive than his own board members about the social policy role he felt business should play.

To identify Goldbeck as important, however, does not deny the fact that other structural factors were crucial in the growth of WBGH. The organization was formed because Roundtable business leaders felt a need for a separate organizational voice on health issues; the American health care "crisis" had made health care costs a public and national issue; and companies had already learned how important health care costs were to their bottom line. Goldbeck stepped in and used these factors to mold the organization to the needs of big business. His vision of how business could and should be involved in public policy may have been the vision of a corporate liberal, but his articulation of these ideas resonated strongly in the business world. He stated the classic big business position in a clear and forceful way, and there were few vocal dissenters. "Business cannot afford to be noncommittal or back away from issues that have immediate financial impact. . . . I believe with a passion that it is possible to take a group of businesses and get them involved in social policy issues. . . . We cannot afford to have that segment absent from the policy debate."[17]

How did Goldbeck and the leaders of the Roundtable plan to involve business in the public policy process in health?

When we began, we laid out a plan that said we would spend two years in strictly awareness building and then four years to get business to create institutions for change. What we really wanted was for big business to become a credible participant in national health policy, so several years from now, no issue will go by without our being a player. We wanted to do this in a way that is dignified—it could have been potatoes, defense, oil, it doesn't matter. If you have a clear objective and a comprehensible process you'll find out quickly if you're right or wrong.

The Washington Business Group on Health, partly because it was organized around a single issue and partly because it had been so closely connected to the Business Roundtable, became very effective in Washington political circles. Its membership had grown steadily since its beginnings with 5 companies in 1974 to 175 in 1980 and a total of almost 200 companies in 1984. By 1988, membership had tapered off to about 180 companies, but the staff and scope of its activities continued to grow.[18] The staff of WBGH grew from one to six in 1983, twelve by 1984, and twenty-six by 1988; the organization was supported by a budget, half of which came from company-paid dues and half from government agencies, foundations, and other organizations. WBGH launched a national journal *Business and Health* in 1983, and a host of programs followed, such as institutes on Rehabilitation and Disability Management; Aging, Work and Health; Organizational Health; the National Center for Mental Health and Work; and the Quality Resource Center.

The membership of the WBGH was technically open to provider groups, but Goldbeck made it clear that WBGH was primarily an organization of purchasers not providers. In 1974, both the AMA and the AHA (American Hospital Association) sat on the advisory committee to WBGH. Ten years later, of the more than 175 members, eight insurance companies, three for-profit hospital chains (American Medical International, National Medical Enterprises, and Hospital Corporation of America), and two drug companies were still members. In spite of the presence of these provider members, Goldbeck talked of the need to break business away from providers. "Our biggest educational step has not been in dealing with business about government, but to break business away from the providers. If there was to be a marker of what we have accomplished, it would be that we have broken down the myths that kept business as a passive purchaser and we have made them aggressive buyers. That is a true change and it will not go away."

Goldbeck felt strongly that business needed to develop its own voice and its own strength in order to affect policy, but he did not and would not ban corporations from membership in WBGH simply because they provided medical service or supplies. He allowed them to be members but continued to emphasize the importance of the purchaser role in health policy, while stating his personal preferences privately:

You give up something when you have all parties working together in these so-called coalitions. You give up any policy role at all. You can work on cost containment to a fare-thee-well but I defy you with all parties present to work effectively on legislation. The future model is to have a business group, just like you have a medical society and a hospital association, and eventually coalitions will be representative of all of these groups at a higher level. But business groups are going to be the dominant change agent. Period.

When Goldbeck spoke for business, not everyone listened. But Capitol Hill committee staff members liked Goldbeck's style because he could play the legislative game and deliver on his promises. He could round up any number of vice presidents or a CEO to speak tò a member of Congress, work on a position paper, make a phone call or write a letter, and even occasionally appear to testify if necessary.

The way that WBGH operated in Washington differed slightly from the Chamber, NAM, or even the Roundtable. Frederick Lee, policy director of WBGH said, "The Business Roundtable influences policy by calling a few people. They don't seek to educate their own members in an aggressive way like we do. We do more than educate business, though. We also educate the community. The Roundtable created WBGH to do its dirty work for it, and now the Roundtable has created a void by not doing some of their dirty work themselves or through their task forces." Goldbeck characterized the difference between the Roundtable and WBGH in a different way. "We do not play the political game at all," said Goldbeck. "We make no political contributions. In ten years I have never taken anybody to lunch. We have never even gone to a political reception."

Goldbeck and his organization were anything if not "political" in the way they wielded influence, however. Goldbeck made it his business to know what was going on with his business constituents, what was going on in Congress, who was up for reelection, and who needed information. He constantly used WBGH as a vehicle for putting people together to discuss long-range policy issues. Not everyone saw WBGH in the same way. David Winston noted, "WBGH's whole reason for existing is to peddle its wares in Washington. That is not the function of the Business

Roundtable. WBGH is there all the time. They're ready and willing to testify on anything at any time. But if the BR wants to testify, somebody has to do it—to prepare it. The BR is not institutionally geared to respond as quickly or frequently and for that reason they may not be called as often."

The issues WBGH chose for the 1980s as major legislative targets are interesting indicators of their strategy: WBGH supported the Tax Equity and Fiscal Responsibility Act of 1982 (TEFRA); the prospective payment system (PPS) for Medicare; Professional Standards Review Organizations (PSROs) and health planning; national disclosure of financial data on hospitals and physicians' patterns of practice; and FTC control over the practice of medicine by the medical profession. WBGH opposed the tax cap and vouchers and remained neutral on state rate setting, although the organization was willing to support whatever local business supported at the state level.

WBGH's policy positions did not all coincide with the Reagan administration's new policy direction. In fact, support for prospective payment was one of the few legislative issues on which WBGH agreed with the administration. These differences, however, did not represent a radical rift. WBGH still supported the market strategy for health policy change and the reinforcement of private control over medical care resources. The dispute caused WBGH more internal than external problems, and it removed them from the inner circle of Reagan policy advisers. According to Goldbeck,

Our toughest issue came up at the beginning of the Reagan administration. Lots of CEOs had promised Reagan and the Party full support for the first budget, no matter what, so that Reagan could turn the economy around. When the first budget came out, there were some glaring inconsistencies we couldn't ignore. The administration wanted to cut out PSROs and health planning, both programs which we as an organization had previously supported. When I prepared to oppose the administration on these issues, some of the members said, "No, you can't. We promised the president." But I just told them we had to be independent, because we would just end up as a political organization. An arm of the Republican party and no more. A few companies left us over the issue.

Although shut out of the executive branch policy-making in health, WBGH did achieve some notable lobbying successes with Congress, some launched from a position of unity within WBGH (e.g., salvaging the Peer Review Organization, financial disclosure and data release, Prospective Payment System, federal waivers) and others from a position of considerable disagreement and debate (e.g., the Federal Trade Commission issue).

WBGH participated aggressively on the financial disclosure and data issue. For example, this leadership could be seen in WBGH's participation and support for employers' access to information about the health care system. WBGH helped Rep. Ron Wyden (R-Ore.) introduce an amendment into a health manpower bill that would give the Department of Health and Human Services (DHHS) the authority to assist business at the state level in their quest for information about the costs of health care. Although it seemed an innocuous issue on its face and sure to pass, both physicians and hospitals lobbied strongly against it, arguing that the data would be difficult to understand and easy to misinterpret by nonprofessionals. WBGH regarded the data and financial disclosure issue as key to its strategy. "Information is power in any situation," said Goldbeck. "And up until recently the providers have kept that information locked away."

The data issue began at the state level and moved to the federal level only after states had passed legislation mandating the disclosure of various types of cost information. Goldbeck immodestly declared, "The data issue wouldn't have existed without WBGH. We cranked up business at the state level and then the federal interest picked up. Congress passed a foot-in-the-door bill, and it passed, but Reagan vetoed it because it was part of a larger bill he opposed. It will come up again. In fact, there is a hearing today [November 18, 1984] over at Senate Appropriations on 'Access to Data.' We were the only business group asked to testify."

Legislation was introduced and eventually passed in 1985 to allow employers to request information from the federal government, and eighteen states had passed financial disclosure laws by the end of 1984 that required providers to give employers information on costs and patterns of practice. Of business and health coalitions reporting to the AHA's 1986–1987 survey, 70.2 percent reported that they were involved in data base activity, and more than 50 percent of the coalitions reporting data activity obtained statewide data from a state data agency, commission, or consortium.[19] By 1988, an increasing number of states had agencies that collected statewide health care data and WBGH had sponsored a National Association of Health Data Organizations, funded by the Hartford Foundation and dedicated to fostering uniformity of data reporting throughout the states.[20] In fact, because of providers' resistance to it, the ownership of information issue, promoted and strongly supported by purchasers, turned out to be an important indicator of the political power of business to effect health policy change.

As WBGH became more effective, it seemed they had to participate less. "The AMA will send car loads of lobbyists up to the Hill on an issue, and we only have to write one note. It's not that we don't ever have to do anything; on some issues like the Federal Trade Commission it took an incredible amount of work. But the more credibility we build up, the less actual appearing we have to do," said Goldbeck, validating the idea that when business does participate it may have more to do with "communicating and reproducing power" than winning or losing on a given policy issue.[21]

The Dunlop Group of Six

Another type of "institutional mechanism" created in the 1980s to influence health policy was the Dunlop Group of Six, a private "club" of the heads of the major stakeholders in health care politics, named after its chairman and convener, Professor John T. Dunlop of Harvard University, a renowned and respected labor negotiator.[22] The Dunlop Group consisted of the heads of the AHA, the AMA, Blue Cross and Blue Shield of America, the commercial insurers (Health Insurance Association of America, HIAA), the national Business Roundtable, and two representatives from labor (the heads of both the AFL-CIO and the Service Employees International Union, SEIU).

The Dunlop Group was formed out of a sense of concern over health care costs and the prospect of either public or private purchaser control of the health care system. Although the business community did not initiate the formation of the Dunlop Group, business provided a major part of the motivation. The vice president of the AMA at the time, Dr. James Sammons, was worried about the impact of business coalitions, primarily because the Chicago business coalition, where the AMA was located, refused to allow medical society members to participate. Sammons was so concerned about what business might do that he instigated a visitation program in the early 1980s in which he, AMA board members, and AMA staff visited 126 Fortune 500 company CEOs and benefit managers. "The Japanese were cleaning our clocks in the 1970s, but CEOs didn't know what they were paying for in health care," remembered Sammons. "We thought we should be the ones to educate them."

In the late 1970s, Sammons and Alexander McMahon, president of the AHA, two old friends from the Wage and Price Control Committee, asked Dunlop to chair a national coalition of the major interests in health care issues to promote the Voluntary Effort in cost containment. This approach to health care cost containment had been proposed by major providers as a way to postpone or avoid some of President Carter's proposals for regulating the cost of health care. The Voluntary Effort failed rather dramatically when health care costs not only increased but also soared in the early 1980s. When Dunlop was originally asked in the late 1970s to pull together the coalition, he was asked to do so as a representative of labor because labor, preferring national health insurance, had refused to participate in the Voluntary Effort. Dunlop refused, too. "If you can't get representatives of labor to work with you, I won't come aboard as their representative," he said.

Sammons and McMahon came back to Dunlop in summer 1980 to ask him to go to labor as well as management leaders and ask them both to participate in a coalition. Dunlop knew just whom to contact. Since 1973, he had chaired the Labor-Management Group for the Business Roundtable, consisting of eight top labor people and eight top CEOs who had a tradition of working together.

When Dunlop asked Lane Kirkland of the AFL-CIO to participate in the "new" coalition, he told him, "You don't have to carry any baggage from the past. The deal is, if you participate, you can maintain all the devotion to national health insurance you want, and we will start from scratch, with no preconceived solutions to problems." Kirkland said yes without hesitation, and he named Bert Seidman as his staff. Walter Wriston of the Business Roundtable also agreed and named Chris York as his staff. Dunlop then met with Jim Morefield of the HIAA and Walter McNerney of Blue Cross, and they both agreed to participate. That gave him his six members. Dunlop insisted that the heads of these associations participate because he felt that the higher up the representation of an organization, the broader the perspective. He also stipulated that representatives to the Dunlop Group would be organizational participants, not individual participants. There could be no commitment without a constituency.

The first year of the Dunlop Group was spent refining a policy statement on developing coalitions and learning how to operate by Dunlop's rules: (1) no one had to abandon his ideology or commitment to long-held goals in order to enter the room; (2) the discussions were to be in private and off the record; and (3) everyone needed to look forward to new ideas.

Dunlop was asked, "Why six members of the Group? Why not seven or eight?" He replied, "We wanted to keep it small and see what agreement we could get with the six." Within a few years, two additional labor representatives were added, John Sweeney of the SEIU and Mel Glasser, representing both the Health Security Action Council and the American Association of Retired Persons (AARP). The addition of labor representatives, most agreed, reflected Dunlop's own commitment to having a strong labor voice in the discussions.

The Dunlop Group was not specifically created by business, nor has it been particularly dominated by business. Why should I include it in a discussion of business institutional mechanisms for change? The Dunlop Group, for the purposes of this discussion, is an important example of the way policy is made and implemented in private. Because the leadership of the major stakeholders, including business, is involved, its process and outcomes deserve some attention. A look at the private, off-the-record process of the Dunlop Group can offer interested observers a sampling of the myriad interactions that influence the policy formation agenda all the time.

What has been the purpose of the Dunlop Group, what does it do in meetings six or seven times a year, and what impact, if any, has it had on the policy process? It is difficult to characterize what the Group does. Although its representatives are clear and even adamant about what they do not do, the evidence is contradictory. The Dunlop Group says it does not endorse legislation; yet Professor Dunlop has carried the message of its members to Washington for behind-the-scenes discussions of pending legislation. The Dunlop Group does not take policy positions; however, it has endorsed the formation and expansion of local business coalitions and published a statement on Medicaid and the uninsured. The Dunlop Group does not deal with issues on which there is substantial policy difference among its members; yet, it has discussed the Kennedy bill for insuring the uninsured and other controversial issues. The Dunlop Group has no particular purpose other than to talk and share ideas with no product in mind; however, it supports the collection of data on business coalitions, publishes position papers, and collects and disseminates health care data.[23] The Dunlop Group could be a powerful force in promoting certain policy agendas, but its members continually and forcefully deny that it has any purpose other than "meeting and talking together."

If the purpose of the Dunlop Group has been publicly confusing, then its process is even more obscure. No person other than "principals," the members themselves or their "dedicated staff," attend the meetings. No formal minutes are kept or distributed, although Dunlop's chief staff person, Galen Young of the AHA, keeps informal notes about the proceedings. The staff to the Group meet between every meeting of the principals to find consensus on issues discussed at the principals' meetings.

How does John Dunlop run a meeting of equals, powerful policy makers in health, and achieve consensus? "Very slowly," said one observer. "He gives an example, sometimes in parable form, and then goes around the room and asks each person what they think. He runs the meetings in concentric circles, zeroing in on matters of consensus, and skillfully avoiding areas of conflict." If there is conflict over an issue (such as medical liability or the taxation of benefits), there would be discussion of the issue for a while because it would not be "gentlemanly" to ignore a member's interest. Most likely, Dunlop would simply talk to that member privately outside the meetings, instead of bringing the conflict back into the Group.

The potential for the purchasers, business and labor, to dominate the

Dunlop Group discussions has been noted but discounted. As one staff member observed, "It's frightening how much business and labor have in common when they get together." Most of the time, however, neither business nor labor pushes its position very strongly. "Don't you [labor and business] have the power to sway opinions within the Group?" the labor representative was asked. "We're not that type of group at all," Bert Seidman of the AFL-CIO responded strongly. "We meet, not to sway, but to exchange positions. It's a very informal group. Low-key." A logical question emerges. Why meet at all if nothing happens, nothing changes? "It's the only place we have to meet where there is no pressure and no particular outcome expected," commented several participants.

What has been the major contribution of business? Galen Young said, "Business has strongly supported alternative delivery systems, but it's amazing how so much power can be exercised [she paused to consider her words] . . . so gently. Business has been almost naive in using their power." In a forum of equals, such as the Dunlop Group, business representatives would seldom have a need to push their agenda aggressively. Moreover, other participants expect that business power is most effective when masked. As political scientist Samuel Huntington has observed, "Effective power is unnoticed. Power observed is devalued."[24]

The conflict between business as purchaser and business as insurer is recognized by all participants of the Group because the business representative to the Group from the national Business Roundtable is also head of a commercial insurance company. When Walter Wriston was the business representative to the Dunlop Group, he represented the power of nonhealth or insurer-related business interests. When Wriston was replaced by John Creedon of the Metropolitan Life Insurance Company in 1985, the overlap of interests between Creedon as insurer and Creedon in his role representing purchasers was not lost on Dunlop himself. "Creedon invited me to a meeting of the Roundtable's health care committee once where I could speak to the 'real' employers," Dunlop commented wryly. Few would claim that commercial insurers are the most effective representatives of big business interests on the Roundtable, but when pressed most members personalized the issue, pointing to John Creedon's scrupulous avoidance of advocacy on issues where there might be a conflict of interest. "If he could not advocate for purchasers unequivocally, he would leave the room," said one participant. "We're aware of the conflicts, and all I can say is that we try our best to be aware of the hat we are wearing," said Nicholas La Trenta, a vice president of Metropolitan Life and staff to Creedon on the Group.

Although the Dunlop Group has undoubtedly helped promote the development and growth of business coalitions around the country through Dunlop's advice to the Robert Wood Johnson Foundation on its coalition program, Community Programs for Affordable Health Care, the collection of data on coalitions, and its open promotion of the coalition idea, its impact on other aspects of health policy is more difficult to assess. It may be important to monitor the activities of the Group in the next few years, particularly the impact of the Group and of the foundations on the growth and survival of business coalitions. Sammons of the AMA observed, "It's probably a good thing that the Robert Wood Johnson Foundation money for coalitions is running out soon because the proof of the pudding is whether coalitions will survive without it."

Business and Health Coalitions

Probably the most visible and dramatic indicator of business interest in health care has been the participation of business in forming and developing hundreds of business and health coalitions in communities around the country. According to some, the response to the failure of public-sector initiatives to control costs in the 1970s was "typically American"; the number, type, and scope of coalitions grew most rapidly from 1982 to 1985 and tapered off in the late 1980s.[25] In 1982, the U.S. Chamber of Commerce counted 25 coalitions around the country, while other estimates placed the number between 60 and 75. Within one year, there were 123 coalitions, and by 1985 there were 173. By 1987, the most reliable count of active operational coalitions was 178.[26] Coalitions became the topic of magazine articles, books, and national surveys, and a source of considerable concern to providers, some of whom regarded them as a threat. Coalitions have been labeled a "third force," a "fourth party," "buyers' cartels," and a "countervailing force." What are these coalitions, who belongs to them, what have they accomplished, and will they last?[27]

Coalitions in health care began to form actively in the late 1970s, although some groups, such as the coalition in Rochester, had worked on health care issues since the late 1960s. According to an AMA spokesman, there were twenty-nine operational coalitions before 1979; according to the AHA/Dunlop Group's numbers, only eight coalitions existed before 1977. Whatever the actual number in the 1970s, it was relatively small, with most estimates giving business the credit for initiating between 40 and 50 percent of these early coalitions.[28] Spurring the development of coalitions in the early 1980s was the intervention and work of the Chamber of Commerce of the U.S., the Washington Business Group on Health, the Labor-Management Group, and all the other organizations already described in this chapter. In addition, several other factors encouraged the development and growth of coalitions: a national policy that had failed to control hospital costs through regulation in the late 1970s;[29] a new administration that was promoting private sector initiatives; a political situation in which "no one group is strong enough, dominant enough, or persuasive enough to dictate policy";[30] an American penchant for the use of informal groups and networks to solve what are perceived as community problems; and, of major importance, the influx of between $10 and $15 million in foundation support for the development of coalitions in the early 1980s.[31]

It has been difficult to report accurate numbers because the coalition's definition is different, depending on the groups that keep the numbers. What is a coalition? It is the most fragile of organizational forms. The Dunlop Group of Six, through the AHA, has the simplest definition: "A health care coalition is a voluntary alliance of discrete interests sharing the principal objective of improving health care cost effectiveness within a community."[32] Goldbeck of WBGH defined it as "an association with purchaser representation whose primary reason is to promote local, rather than national, health care cost containment efforts."[33] The Chamber of Commerce directory only solicited information from groups that met three criteria: significant representation by nonhealth businesses as purchasers of care; a list of members submitted to the Clearinghouse to document membership; and some sort of cost-containment strategy begun or near implementation. The Dunlop/AHA directory had no requirement that there be significant representation of nonhealth businesses; in fact, the whole purpose of the AHA effort was to encourage multipurpose coalitions and discourage employer or business-only coalitions.[34]

The AHA also required that the coalition be an established group and in the process of implementing programs to be considered operational. The number of coalitions that could be counted as operational at any given time, however, depended on the response rate to the various surveys. When the AHA data base was evaluated by a team from the Robert Wood Johnson (RWJ) Foundation in 1987 all 215 coalitions previously listed as active by the AHA were called by the evaluators; 37 were found inactive or dissolved by late 1987, leaving 178 active and operational coalitions in early 1987.

More important than the actual number of coalitions were other issues about coalitions: Who would maintain the national data base on coalitions? How many employer-only coalitions really existed? What impact might they have on health care policy? And what differences, if any, did these coalitions make at the local level? The power over the data base was resolved in 1985, when the Chamber of Commerce ceased publishing its Clearinghouse directory and gave the responsibility for keeping track of health care coalitions to the AHA/Dunlop Group. The Washington Business Group on Health wanted to participate as keeper of the numbers, but the funding went to the AHA.

Who won or lost on this issue is significant mainly in terms of the attitudes of these various groups toward counting business or employer-only coalitions. Professor Dunlop had a clear agenda for promoting multiparty coalitions. Although he stated publicly and privately that he did not object to the formation or existence of business-only coalitions, he also repeatedly emphasized that the problems could be solved only through collaborative action. Dunlop's philosophy was reflected in the way the numbers were kept by the AHA. By 1988, the AHA directory counted only 9.3 percent "business-only" coalitions, while the RWJ evaluators found that 45 percent of the coalitions in the same data base identified themselves as business-only. The discrepancy occurred in counting voting and nonvoting members. "A member is not a member is not a member," noted one evaluator.[35] If a coalition reported that business members were voting members but that provider members were "nonvoting associates," the AHA counted them as multiparty coalitions, while the coalitions themselves and the RWJ evaluators counted them as business-only.

Why would Dunlop and the providers take such pains to characterize these coalitions as multiparty? What was the threat of a business-only coalition? The providers had their own associations. Why should business not have its own? One problem with the battle over coalition structure was the origin of the coalition. About half the coalitions around the country had been initiated by business, many of them as adjunct organizations to already existing business groups or associations. The providers could do nothing to control the existence of a local or statewide business roundtable, but when the roundtable began to establish task forces to consider health issues the providers felt they should be part of the discussion. A conflict over ownership and leadership of the health care coalitions resulted.

Business members and provider members viewed the purpose and utility of a coalition in different ways. The purchasers viewed business-only coalitions as opportunities for business members to exchange information. "We find that exchange of information is always a little more free when people feel that they are operating in a peer group," said the president of the nine-state Midwest Business Group on Health.[36] Business also regarded the coalition structure as a way to develop bargaining strategies for use with providers. Chris York, vice president of Citibank and member of the Dunlop Group, commented, "When we sit down in September to plan how many typewriters we are going to order, we do not have the equipment sales representative sitting in that little collegial budget meeting. That does not mean we hate him; indeed, we want to maintain cordial relationships with him."[37] To business, it was not a matter of like or dislike; it was a business relationship between producer and seller. Lee Iacocca of the Chrysler Corporation noted, "What you have is a huge vested interest, the doctors and the hospitals, that says this is a profession, this isn't a supplier, and you keep your cotton-picking hands off. If I want to buy steel, I can go to the lowest seller, but in health, the buyer-seller relationship doesn't exist. Yet, in fact, Blue Cross/Blue Shield is my biggest supplier."[38]

The physician community continued to hold an entirely different perspective on the process. Charles Marcus, executive director of the Colorado Medical Society, said, "Having a coalition of business people without physicians is like putting together physicians to discuss how to manufacture automobiles."[39] The professionals strongly believed that decisions in health care could only be resolved by those technically competent in the field. By defining the issue this way, physicians characterized this conflict as a straightforward clash between professional and managerial control. "A major tension at the core of professionalism is the conflicting pressure stemming from the relationship between occupational authority on the one hand and consumer choice on the other." Although big business in no way wished to deny physicians their technical expertise, they certainly intended to define its boundaries within their own managerial domain.[40]

Both the threat of conflict between purchasers and providers and the possibility of the effective exercise of purchasing power had been pervasive concerns throughout the provider community from the beginning of the coalition movement. The articles on business coalitions were filled with references to these threats by the business community to use their power. For example, when the Arizona business coalition took on the hospital association in a series of ballot initiatives designed to regulate hospital costs in 1984, *Business Week* called it "high noon in Arizona for hospitals costs," and the hospitals called it "all-out corporate warfare."[41] Robert Burnett, CEO of the Meredith Corporation, told his fellow corporate officers, "Initially, we attempted to effect change through negotiation, discussion, debate, through participation of all of the interests with a vested economic stake in health care delivery. I know what the arguments are for using a more conciliatory approach because I accepted them and sought—unsuccessfully, I might add—to effect change through this route. . . . I am now convinced that we should have been more aggressive . . . and willing to insist upon quicker responses and faster action."[42] George Murphy, president of San Diego's Community Health Care Alliance, noted, "When the coalition was created, the providers were concerned that employers were forming a health care purchasing cartel which would own them lock, stock and barrel."[43]

Not all providers were eager to negotiate with business. Steven Seiler, president of Lake Forest Hospital, remembers that when the Employers' Health Care Group of Lake County, Illinois, was incorporated in 1980 and attempted to negotiate with the hospitals, "the reaction of the hospitals was something akin to the Mount Saint Helens eruption."[44] According to Seiler, the hospitals finally were drawn into negotiating with the major employers for several reasons: (1) they realized that the employer group was not going to disappear; (2) the companies involved in the coalition would ultimately use their connections as trustees of hospital boards to bring pressure on the hospitals to cooperate; and (3) the hospitals could best protect their interests by being at the table with the coalition. In Illinois where John Deere and Caterpillar are dominant employers, Seiler noted, "The relationship is clearly adversarial."

In this atmosphere of differing goals and strategies, it was to the providers' benefit to construct the issue as one in which conflict would be dangerous. However, not only providers but also business people sought to avoid controversy. In fact, very few business participants wished to become involved in a situation that would pit them against their local institutions and the power of the medical profession in their community. Big business may have had substantial market power, but the barriers to unleashing it were equally substantial.

The relationship between conflict and consensus is critical in U.S. politics. Seymour Lipset has noted that a major area within political sociology is the study of the balance between conflict and consensus. Samuel Huntington has further commented, "In the American experience, consensus is not an alternative to political conflict, but is, rather, a source of political conflict."[45] Health policy observers have noted that the interaction between conflict and consensus is complex but necessary in health care politics. "Coalitional activities should be done with a civil spirit of negotiation and compromise; strategies should be guided by a sense of community. Still . . . no truly innovative project can succeed on a consensus basis. Instead the coalition approach requires tough leadership by the committed."[46]

Not only do employers and providers hold distinctly different views on the purpose of coalitions, but they are also considerably divergent in their views on the importance and viability of the various cost-containment initiatives proposed by coalitions. A poll by Louis Harris and Associates in 1983 found that 79 percent of corporate benefits officers agreed with the statement that "there are some good things in our health care system, but fundamental changes are needed to make it work better," while only 56 percent of hospital administrators and 32 percent of physician leaders agreed with the same statement. Corporate benefit officers and insurers also were more likely to advocate cost control than were hospitals or physicians, with physicians railing against government regulation, an issue employers found of little or no importance.[47]

With so much activity over the potential threat of exercising business power, the actual accomplishments of some business coalitions have been obscured. One survey of 122 Business Roundtable corporations found that 90 percent of the companies participated in health care coalitions and nearly 80 percent encouraged such participation as a corporate policy.[48] But what were the outcomes? The major issues of interest for coalitions by 1988, along with cost containment, were quality of care, financing uncompensated care, medical professional liability, mandated health benefits, and retiree health benefits.[49] The most prevalent activities of most coalitions were education of its members, data collection, benefit design, alternative delivery system development, legislative analysis and advocacy, and health promotion and wellness. Several studies have noted that business-only coalitions were more likely to engage in active interventions in the health care system, such as the design of alternative delivery systems, data gathering and interpretation, and legislative advocacy, while multiparty coalitions were often stuck at the level of educating their members.[50]

Whether community coalitions have been successful in actually containing costs within the community has not yet been documented and is hotly debated. The head of the Midwest Business Group of Health reported in 1987, "There is increasing evidence that in a competitive health care marketplace, the community-based, voluntary, multidiscipline approach to health care problem-solving is no longer workable."[51] In fact, the number of operational coalitions was declining by the end of the 1980s, suggesting a number of alternative hypotheses: This organizational form had not satisfied the cost-containment objectives of the business community; other vehicles were being sought for leverage on the system; business representatives were getting tired of so many cost-containment lunches; or the decline was temporary and likely to change as costs began to increase again.[52]

The RWJ evaluation report of twenty-one community coalitions was intended to produce some of the first evidence of actual impact on community health care costs. Meanwhile, the preliminary conclusions were not very positive. The evaluators concluded, "Our findings cast doubt on the hypothesis that a broad assemblage of community elites, led by such voluntary institutions as Blue Cross and Blue Shield and hospitals, can sustain negotiating processes that yield effective leadership in containing costs."[53] They noted that several forces were inhibiting the sustained effectiveness of these coalitions: First, variables that determine costs do not generally lie within the community's grasp so the community may not be the most powerful locus of leadership in health care cost containment. Second, even if the community were a plausible setting, most local power structures would be unable to generate the leadership required, that is, there is not a sufficient concentration of power in the hands of most purchasers to force change. And third, negotiations among community elites on local projects will not yield promising outcomes because the balloon of health care costs is only being squeezed on one end. A more promising site for health care reform would be found at the state or national level.

The number of business coalitions appears to have developed, grown, and tapered off throughout the 1980s, primarily as a result of the need for a mechanism by business for information and leverage on the health care system. As the first generation of solutions fails to control costs completely or as information becomes available from other sources, some need for coalitions will disappear. However, even if these coalitions change their goals or structure or go out of business in the 1990s, their disappearance will not invalidate their existence in the 1980s as legitimate, although temporary, institutional mechanisms for change. These coalitions have provided business interests a credible and sometimes effective mechanism for expressing business interests in health care politics.

The power of business in the policy process is demonstrated by its ability to articulate its interests through just such organizations as the Chamber or the WBGH and to translate that interest into legislative action. What began as a concern by government in the late 1960s about medical care costs was picked up by a few members of the dominant segment of the American business elite in the early 1970s. These concerns were carried through and between the various elite policy organizations and resulted in the creation of new organizations formed in the mid-1970s. By the time Reagan was elected president in 1980, some top business leaders were reasonably aware of the problems, and business had several institutional mechanisms through which to respond. The fact that the business community itself was still divided and did not necessarily support all Reagan cost-containment proposals should not obscure the fact that most proposals increased the power of the private sector to finance and deliver medical care and that the competitive marketplace approach to health policy change was itself in great part promoted by business policy groups in the 1970s.

By the late 1980s, with a few institutional mechanisms in place, the largest American corporations had declared their intention to play a stronger role in the health policy process at all levels of government, through participation in coalitions, alliances, and state and federal commissions and advisory bodies. There were some differences between small and big business; small business tended to support more competitive, market policies, and big business tended to support regulation. And older manufacturing and banking industries and high technology business likewise differed in approach; the more stable manufacturing industries and banks were more willing to participate politically in the communities where their headquarters were located, and high technology was more likely to simply move a plant when costs got too high. But business as a purchaser had declared itself to have a political interest in affecting health policy. Business created institutional mechanisms for change, some permanent and others less so, to promote its interest in the national health policy debate.

5

The Federal Context:
A Wedge of
Structural Change

JUST AS THE CREATION of Medicare and Medicaid in the 1960s had stimulated private-sector changes, federal policy initiatives in the Medicare
and Medicaid programs between 1980 and 1982 created a window of opportunity for state health policy changes in both private and public sectors for the remainder of the 1980s. Many factors at the national level
provided the context within which business could more effectively participate and affect policy: *the ideology of policy* in the Reagan administration and the way in which certain agendas and interests dominated the
policy process; *the interaction of state structures* over certain policies
and the way decisions were fragmented among various bureaucratic
agencies; and the *readiness of business elites* to become involved in
forming a policy agenda that would promote structural change in the
health care sector.

The Ideology of Policy Change

In 1980, some Reagan administration changes in health policy affected all levels of government. None of these dramatic ideas was particularly new, not even "new" Federalism. What was surprising to the
political actors themselves was the speed with which some of these ideas
were accepted and implemented into law and the degree to which the
policy debate shifted from a preoccupation with regulation and national
health insurance in the 1970s to the obsession with the market approach
to policy change in the 1980s.

It is difficult to determine what role party and leadership played in accepting these policy ideas and to what degree economic, historical, and other political conditions predisposed the system to change. Certainly the growth of medical technology, the bureaucratization and increasing corporatization of health care organizations, rising health care costs, economic recession and fiscal crisis, the weakening of professionals as individual entrepreneurs, and even the international debt crisis all contributed to the crisis of reform. How the system changed—to what degree and in what direction—can be most accurately explained by the way in which strategic elites in the Reagan administration took advantage of a cycle of crisis and reform, leading to further crisis, that had gripped the American health care system for almost fifteen years. Instead of playing the usual pluralist game of incremental, marginal, and largely symbolic changes, the Reagan policy makers went for the "big win" and what has been called the "thin end of the wedge of structural change."[1]

Each of Reagan's new ideas could be traced to the Nixon administration, including the reliance on competition through the stimulation of HMOs, the antiregulation stance, budget cuts in health and human service programs, and block grants to the states. Even the new prospective payment system, different incentives for provider behavior, and government as "prudent purchaser" ideas could be found in thought and action of earlier decades.[2] However, coupled with the powerful ideological commitment to competition in all areas of American industry within the Reagan administration, the promotion of competition in health care was given extra potency.

The strength of the market ideology was further assured by the almost religious fervor of the health policy advocates within the Reagan administration. As Canadian health economist Robert Evans has observed of American health policy, "The free market is not preferred because it achieves other objectives, whether of cost, quality or access; it is *itself* the objective. . . . This normative position . . . is not merely intellectually isomorphic with religion, it *is* a religion."[3] A defense of the market as allocator of resources comes from Clark Havighurst, a health economist who was active on Reagan's first health policy advisory group. Havighurst extols "rationing care through market choices rather than through governmental mechanisms" because tragic choices such as who will live and who will die "need not [be made] through the already overburdened political process."[4]

One of the earliest documents outlining what would become the direction of the Reagan administration's initiatives in health policy was the November 14, 1980, memorandum from the Health Policy Advisory Group, or the Walsh Group as it would be called, to President-elect Ronald Reagan.[5] The nation's prominent conservative health economists, market-oriented Republican members of Congress, provider interest groups, including a strong representation from drug manufacturers, and the Ford Motor Company all participated in drafting the memorandum. Their recommendations provided a base for future policy advisory groups and incorporated the general principles of what would come to be known as the Reagan agenda: procompetition (the basic elements of which were increased consumer choice, tax policy that stimulates choice, and placing providers at risk); altered government's role as regulator for a few people to buyer and subsidizer; decentralized decision making from federal to state and local levels; and changed incentives for both buying and selling health care by government, consumers, and business. The report advocated continuing the voluntary effort by providers to bring down costs and even mentioned the stimulation of local cost containment coalitions among business, labor, providers, and local governments. The authors recommended that "assistance [to business coalitions] should be in the form of education and proselytizing."

Barely seven months into the new administration's term, the newly appointed secretary of Health and Human Services, former congressman Richard Schweiker, had already begun to implement many suggestions proposed by the Walsh Group through forming an internal advisory group of his own. Former congressman David Stockman had become director of the Office of Management and Budget (OMB) and was promoting his own version of a conservative health policy agenda. These events led John Iglehart, editor of the prestigious *New England Journal of Medicine,* to note, "If his [Stockman's] views are implemented, they will lead to radical changes in the existing medical order."[6]

The way in which Reagan's policy agenda items were moved along the policy "assembly line" indicates the way in which elites institutionalize ideas that finally gain dominance in the policy decision-making process. As are most such circles, the health policy inner circle was rather small: a few conservative think tank economists; provider groups such as the for-profit hospital association—the Federation of American Hospitals (FAH), the AHA, the AMA; Blue Cross and commercial insurers; the pharmaceutical industry; and certain former members of Congress and their staff. Members of the original transition team (for example, David Stockman, Richard Schweiker, Donald Moran, and Schweiker's former staff member David Winston) were appointed to high-level positions, hired as staff members within the federal health bureaucracy, or reappointed to succeeding policy task force groups.

One such group working concurrently with Schweiker's task force was the Private Sector Task Force on Competition, later dubbed the Winston task force because of its leader David Winston, then vice president of Blythe Eastman Paine Webber Health Care Funding, Inc., an important capital funding source for hospital corporations. The Winston task force was created as an adjunct to the HHS internal task force and was part of the administration strategy to "obtain the support or at least the neutrality of key provider groups."[7]

The Winston task force included all the types of stakeholders in the Walsh Group, plus representatives of legal firms specializing in health care litigation, nursing schools, Kaiser Foundation, and two representatives of business, Jack Shelton of the Ford Motor Company, and Chris York, vice president of Citibank, New York.[8] The task force members were mostly Winston's friends, chosen for their pragmatism and flexibility. They met for about seven months, but the road to consensus was not smooth. A few months prior to releasing the task force report in January 1982, to the chagrin of the administration, several task force members testified at a House Ways and Means hearing against the major elements of the administration's competitive proposals, including a tax on employee benefits and a voucher plan for Medicare. The list of opposition to the administration was much longer than the list of supporters, and the final report was only three months away.

In the next three months, a great deal of behind-the-scenes maneuvering took place, including President Reagan's meeting with physicians from the AMA and Schweiker's meetings with key members of the provider community. The administration threatened either a competitive or a regulatory solution, both of which were opposed by various provider interests, but not the status quo. As a result of the bargaining among interests and the pressure from the White House, the final report of the Winston task force managed to achieve temporary consensus echoing the three main themes of the Walsh report: New Federalism, private financing and delivery of health care, and competition.[9]

The task force recommended several new proposals that became critically important for state and private-sector policy changes a year later: a shift from a proposed tax cap on employers to one on employee-paid health premiums; vouchers for Medicare and authority for states to contract for group coverage of Medicaid eligibles; prospective payment for hospitals reimbursed by Medicare; elimination of health planning and the PSROs; multiple choice options for employees in private companies that would promote but not mandate selection of preferred provider organizations and health maintenance organizations. Most of these changes, except the tax cap, were implemented in some form or other by the mid-1980s, and all represented substantial changes in health policy direction.

The Reagan health agenda had been proclaimed within a year of his inauguration through documents such as the Winston report, but no comprehensive competitive bill was introduced into Congress by the end of 1981. For the first six months in 1982, action at the national legislative level was almost completely stalled, while interest groups and the bureaucratic agencies maneuvered for positional advantage.

While Washington fiddled with its grand ideas about competition, the states burned. The worst recession in ten years had made its impact on state budgets. Seven states ended FY 1981–1982 with a deficit, and only twelve reported a surplus of more than 5 percent.[10] Meanwhile, health policy action at the state level grew to a frenzied peak. Between January and June 1982 Massachusetts and California took advantage, not of federal legislation because there was none, but of federal administrative changes that allowed both states to restructure their Medicaid programs by applying federally approved waivers and relaxing previously rigid federal policies on freedom of choice of providers and contracting. Although targeted to the public sector, these policy changes resulted in opportunities for the private sector as well. The public sector door was opened a crack, and an army of private-sector entrepreneurs eventually stormed through.

State Structures: The Bureaucracy and the Congress

It would be a mistake to concentrate on the special interests, private-sector advisory groups, and their agenda for change without paying attention to the congressional committees and bureaucratic agencies. HHS and OMB, along with various House and Senate members and their staff, all played an important role in shaping and pushing the national policy agenda through the committee and budget reconciliation process. In early 1981, the competition legislation was moving slowly in the legislative pipeline because of internal disagreements and turf arguments between Schweiker's people at HHS and Stockman's people at OMB, as well as opposition from the Democratically controlled House of Representatives. Stockman and Schweiker were locked in a personal and departmental power struggle, with Stockman winning most disputes; bills were being introduced at an astonishing rate only to be bogged down in congressional committees; and furious debates were being held over issues that clearly had no chance of passing the 1981 Congress (for example, the tax cap, opposed by almost everyone, especially business, which had begun to mobilize against the issue).

The Omnibus Reconciliation Act (OBRA) of 1981, when it finally passed, did more than just reconcile opposing points of view into a colorless compromise. OBRA actually made substantial policy changes—changes that released state legislatures and health departments from a whole series of constraints on the management of their Medicaid programs and paved the way for a prospective payment system for Medicare. The changes in state Medicaid programs were of significant interest to more knowledgeable business participants because of the real and potential cost shifts from the public to the private sector at the state level. The recommendation that the HHS secretary study prospective payment by the following year was the sleeper policy change of the decade. The fact that both these changes were inserted into the omnibus budget act meant that special interest groups did not have their usual access to the policy process. Business did not fare poorly under OBRA, however, despite its complaints about being shut out of the process. "The OBRA of 1981 represented the most sweeping implementation of employer priorities in the history of the unemployment insurance program. Though it did not exhaust the employers' wish list of unemployment-related cuts, it did meet the employers' demands to a greater extent than had previously been thought possible."[11]

OBRA of 1981 may have been bad budget policy on the part of the Congress, but it was brilliant health policy. The use of the budget as an agent of change became firmly entrenched in 1981 congressional politics. Both bureaucrats and lawmakers realized that they could use the budget as a Trojan horse, filling it with controversial proposals that special interests could not defeat.

Meanwhile, back in Washington, the administration was still frustrated over its failure to pass a major competition bill in the first term. In March 1982, Professor Alain Enthoven of Stanford, a member of the transition team on health policy, blasted the administration for its "retreat from competition." The White House, stung by his criticism, let it be known through Ed Meese that they were looking for a "health czar" to push through their program.[12]

What the White House got was not a czar. California had their Medi-Cal Czar, but Washington got David Winston.[13] Winston was not a mover and a shaker. He was a loyalist. He had been with Reagan in California, a member of the California Assembly budget committee, and had worked in Washington as a staff member in both the Senate and the House, but he had recently returned to private-sector work. Winston agreed to devote two days a week to come up with a proposal that would be politically acceptable to all the interests within sixty days of July 19, 1982. He went back again to each interest group with whom he had met so extensively the previous year and tried to get their support for a way to reduce health care costs without regulation. He would ask, "What do you think ought to be in this package?" And the answer was always the same. Little or nothing in the way of positive ideas. After six weeks there were no new ideas and no changes in positions.

When Ed Harper at the White House asked Winston what he had for them, Winston replied, "I have a long list of groups opposed to competition [that is, tax caps and vouchers], an even longer list of those ambivalent about it; and a short list of those we can count on to be supportive." Those groups opposed to tax caps and vouchers were commercial insurers, labor, physicians, and all the business groups, the ambivalent groups included the hospitals and Blue Cross; the supportive group included only the for-profit hospitals, the health industry manufacturers, and the pharmaceutical industry. Winston's final proposal contained the same ideas his task force had suggested the year before, with the addition of stronger support for prospective payment among some interests. Winston had done all he could.

With 1982 designated as the "year of the states," it is noteworthy that any national health care legislation passed at all. But the administration, mainly Schweiker and HHS, had submitted a budget that included eight proposals affecting Medicaid (all legislative) and sixteen affecting Medicare (ten legislative and six administrative). All had been proposed or discussed in the various task forces or on the Hill; most were defeated by Congress, but cuts in both Medicaid and Medicare programs passed, embedded in the 1982 budget bill, the Tax Equity and Fiscal Responsibility Act (TEFRA) of 1982. TEFRA would be remembered for requiring the secretary to develop a prospective payment system for Medicare, not just a study as mandated in 1982. Four months after the system was reported to Congress, in April 1983, prospective payment and the DRG concept (that is, paying hospitals based on diagnosis related groups of disease) were law. [14]

The idea of prospective payment had been mentioned in the Walsh Group's proposals, the Winston task force recommendations, and Winston's informal meetings with special interests. Schweiker had placed prospective payment at the top of his list of ideas that could and should be implemented, even during the frenetic spring of 1982. The AHA had been supporting prospective payment although on a per discharge basis; the FAH joined them in June 1982. Despite the haste with which it passed and the opposition of physicians, the groundwork for the passage of prospective payment had been carefully laid since the late 1970s.

With the federal government becoming a prudent purchaser, the private sector was not at all far behind. Changes that both OBRA and TEFRA had made regarding tax incentives for investor-owned corporations would, along with DRGs, spur the greatest growth in the for-profit sector of health care that the country had ever seen. Most business leaders were not against profit for the medical care industry and not opposed to the growth of the for-profit sector, although there were some murmurs about increased costs to business if the for-profit industry successfully shifted costs and patients back to the public sector.

By the end of Reagan's first term, the ideology that had dominated the policy debates in the early years of the administration had become entrenched, although implementing these policy ideas had had mixed success. Competition was to be preferred over regulation, unless regulation significantly contained costs. State-level policy change was preferred over federal control, except when states backslide as in the case of Arizona, where business favored regulation.[15] Private-sector initiatives were favored over public-sector domination, except that the federal government was one of the most powerful initiators of change with its DRG system. Behavior change through voluntary market incentives was favored over mandatory regulation, except that David Stockman wanted to be able to overrule states that did not support administration policy.

Within this inconsistent general framework, specific proposals such as vouchers, tax caps, and elimination of federal planning and review programs were largely defeated. States, reacting to the new ideological climate in Washington that encouraged "state discretion," had already begun to take action. In the early 1980s, forty states reduced their Medicaid spending by cutting benefits or lowering payments to providers, sixteen states instituted copayments for some services, and fourteen states reduced the number of eligible beneficiaries. Thirty-three states sought federal waivers for some aspect of their Medicaid program, although sixteen states used the new flexibility to increase the size and scope of their Medicaid programs by adding new services or reinstating previous cuts. The trend in the late 1980s was to augment, not reduce Medicaid, particularly for women and children.[16]

By the beginning of Reagan's second term in 1985, health care costs had begun to rise again, but no comprehensive competition bill was ever introduced. Health care costs would be left to the states to negotiate on behalf of public recipients and to the corporations to negotiate on behalf of covered workers. The increasing number of uninsured Americans, estimated by some to be thirty-seven million by the end of the decade, would be dealt with first at the state level, as happened in Massachusetts. No national solution to the uninsured was in sight by the end of 1988. The Medicare Catastrophic Coverage Act, passed by the Congress and signed by President Reagan in June 1988, expanded Medicare coverage somewhat, but it did not solve the problems of insuring nursing home care for the elderly, and the elderly revolted against it.

The Role of Business in Federal Policy Change

Just as the state-level policy changes could not have occurred without the opening wedge of federal policy initiatives, neither is it likely that local business would have become as involved without the leadership and participation of national business leaders and their organizations. As I have discussed in Chapter 4, throughout the 1970s, business was educating its leadership and creating institutional mechanisms for policy change. When the Reagan administration created its policy task forces and asked for input on the competition proposals, prominent business members were always included. John Harper of Alcoa, Walter Wriston of Citibank/Citicorp of New York, and Henry Ford, Jr., were informed and often participated. These were not just any three business representatives, however; each had been actively involved in the influential Committee for Economic Development discussions in the early and mid-1970s, and they had served on the health care task force of the Business Roundtable. Walter Wriston had turned down President Reagan's invitation to be Treasury secretary in order to be chairman of the Business Council. Of course, issues of deregulation, government spending, and tax reform were much higher on the national business agenda than health care reform at the beginning of the 1980s, which may explain why Chris York was sent to the Winston Group instead of Walter Wriston. Nevertheless, interest in and knowledge of health policy at the level of this type of corporation guaranteed that the voice of business would be heard.

Representatives of big business had some reason to believe that health policy alternatives would be chosen by the Reagan administration that would be consistent with their interests. Except for the few policies described in the previous chapter where business input was important in defeating the power of physicians, their participation was not heavily required at the national level. Instead, all the national business organizations supported the development of local- and state-level business initiatives and coalitions on health. An even greater degree of activity was occurring within corporations, as managers learned they could save money by restructuring benefit programs and shifting more costs to employees.[17] The 1980s saw an increased attention paid in the business press to company-specific strategies to contain health care costs; new journals and magazines devoted specifically to business and health; conferences and forums held around the country to educate business; and new state-level legislation that would give business the information resources through which to exercise its purchasing power at the state and local level.

Although not every aspect of Reagan's market ideology benefited every sector of business, the major policy direction in the early 1980s was consistent with larger purchaser interests to the extent that these policy changes:

1. preserved the power of the private sector over financing and delivering medical care (almost no business representatives were advocating national health service or national health insurance in the early 1980s);

2. increased the purchasing power of the private sector and gave business more control over politics;

3. increased the legitimacy of state power and forced the state to act more as a "prudent buyer" for its own constituencies, the poor and the elderly, which had the potential, if not the reality, of moderating the cost shifts from the public to the private sector;

4. "rationalized" the medical care economy to a greater degree (that is, organized the economy, so that both health-related and non-health-related corporations could function in a more predictable and secure environment);

5. encouraged the flow of capital to the Sunbelt and the large for-profit corporations, and through a greater corporatization of medical care, disciplined the individual institutions and entrepreneurs of the medical care industry;

6. stabilized cost increases in the acute care sector of the medical care industry;

7. shifted costs from management to labor wherever possible and developed liaisons between business and the state by means of commissions and other types of planning bodies to buffer corporations from negative labor reaction and anticipated potential unrest.

When Reagan's second term had ended in 1988, the impact of federal health policies had temporarily slowed the growth of health care costs. The one policy change most opposed by business and other interests, the tax cap on employer-paid premiums, had been roundly defeated, despite the enthusiasm of conservative economists for the idea. The change from retrospective to prospective reimbursement for Medicare, an accelerated shift in federal role from regulator to prudent buyer, and increased discretionary authority at the state level promised substantial structural changes in the health care delivery system. Business support for these changes strengthened the alliance of business and the state, as I will describe in Chapters 6 and 7.

6

Crabs in a Bucket:
Business and Health Policy
Change in California

IN 1982 AS A RESULT of federal policy initiatives and state fiscal crisis, an epidemic of Medicaid policy changes erupted throughout the states. By dint of statute (OBRA of 1981 and TEFRA of 1982) and ideology (decentralized federal and increased private-sector responsibility), the Reagan administration encouraged each state to develop its own response to the growing costs of state Medicaid programs. Many states, including California and Massachusetts, passed legislation intended to dramatically curtail Medicaid costs and restructure Medicaid programs within the state.

At a medical society meeting in a coastal California town in 1983, several physicians were discussing the potential impact of the state legislation passed in 1982. "We're like crabs in a bucket," said one. "Do you know what happens to crabs when you put them in a bucket together?" He paused dramatically and announced, "They EAT each other!"[1]

The legislation that called for this dramatic metaphor was AB 799 and AB 3480 (MediCal reform).[2] When fully implemented, it was intended to introduce price competition among physicians and hospitals and change the incentives to seek, deliver, and finance health care in both the public and private sectors in California. These two bills established negotiated contracting by the state and private insurers with hospitals and physicians and transferred the responsibility for treating 275,000 medically indigent adults (MIAs) from the state to the counties. This combination of reprivatizing financing and shifting public health responsibility to a lower level of government was made possible through a successful challenge to physicians by an active coalition of government, business, labor, insurance, and senior citizens (the Roberti Coalition),[3] and a passively resistant and divided hospital association. Some claim that this active coalition strengthened the autonomous policy capacity of the state, permanently fragmenting both physician and hospital management interests in health care. Some political observers even called it a "revolution" in health care politics.[4]

What happened in California in 1982, whether or not a revolution, was definitely not an isolated attempt at health policy change. While California and Arizona were experimenting with market approaches to policy change, in Massachusetts a similar coalition of business and insurance interests forced the hospitals and physicians to come to terms with a more "regulatory" approach (see Chapter 7).[5] Both Maine and Wisconsin passed rate-setting legislation between 1982 and 1984. Thus California's efforts in 1982 were part of a nationwide trend of health policy change at the state level, stimulated in part by the federal policy initiatives discussed in Chapter 5 and in part by business participation and interest in health policy change. Some might say California was "out in front"; others just "out of step."[6]

This chapter makes two main points: First, the role of business in the passage of this legislation indicates its increasing strength as an active participant in the politics of health policy change at the state level. This exercise of business power had an impact on the political process in California and has had a continuing impact on labor and the autonomy of physicians. Second, the political process that resulted in this legislation is a key to understanding the altered power relationships in California health politics. It can be argued that the power of the dominant providers' interests was reduced through internal fragmentation and the emergence of other equally powerful interests. Such a change has important implications for the balance of power in the health care system and the possibilities for future policy change.

Until 1982, when business interests became active participants in the political process of health policy change in California, hospitals and physicians had always been treated as the most powerful interests by policymakers. This case offers the opportunity to analyze the emerging alliance of the state with business interests, an alliance that had substantial impact on both the balance of political power among special interests and the way in which health policy issues were defined.

The Economic and Political Context for Policy Change

In passing AB 799 and AB 3480, the major policy bills, California legislators were reacting to a series of economic crises in the state. By the end of 1981, a combination of rising costs and falling state revenue pushed the legislators toward action.[7] The fabled $3.7 billion state budget surplus of 1978, which had stimulated the passage of Proposition 13, had been all but used up. A deepening general economic recession was placing pressure on state welfare expenditures at the same time that tax revenues were falling to unprecedented levels. Local county reserves had been depleted through the loss of the federal revenue sharing programs. Between 1978 and 1982, California moved from having one of the nation's highest ratios of taxes to personal income to a position near the median of all states. This was prompted not only by Proposition 13 but also by income tax indexing.[8] Federal cutbacks in block grants (FY1982 decrease of 9.3 percent) and cutbacks in Medicare and Medicaid programs in 1980–1981 threatened the already precarious state funding of the California Medicaid program, MediCal. In this general fiscal crisis, the rising costs of health care in California were especially dramatic. Medical inflation had been about 15 to 18 percent per year (about double the rate of general inflation). As a result of the passage of the OBRA of 1981, California was going to lose 3 percent of the federal match for its Medicaid program in 1982–1983 (an estimated loss of $42.8 million in 1982 and $82 million in 1983). In addition, California had one of the most generous Medicaid programs in the country, with benefits that even included acupuncture. The "working poor" or MIAs were covered entirely by state funds, with no federal matching contribution.[9]

Every year since 1971, the legislature had been asking the Department of Health Services to "do something about MediCal," but those incremental alterations had produced no substantial savings to the state. Critics charged that these policy changes did nothing to alter the perverse incentives in the system, that rewarded acute care over home care, emergency rooms over the doctor's office, and cost shifts from public to private patients. In 1978 State Senator John Garamendi (D, Walnut Grove), a long-time advocate of health system reform, had introduced legislation embodying substantial changes in the MediCal system (SB 716). Among other things, his bill proposed that the Department of Health Services contract on a prospective basis with hospitals for treating MediCal patients. It was roundly defeated and, according to Garamendi, was called "communistic" and "un-American" by the California Medical Association (CMA).

The CMA could just as easily have attacked hospital contracting on the basis of its mixed record in California. In the early 1970s under the Reagan administration in California, several attempts were made to bring MediCal eligibles into HMOs, and the state tried contracting with nonprofit health care organizations. The resulting scandals and mismanagement damaged the reputation of contracting and prepaid group plans for the next decade, at least as solutions to caring for the poor.[10]

In 1981, desperate for a workable solution, the California legislature succeeded in passing a variation of Garamendi's 1978 proposal. AB 251 contained several precursors of the 1982 policy changes, including contracting by the state with hospitals on a pilot basis, primary case management, and a transfer of MIAs into county health systems. This legislation was projected to save $85.5 million from the state general fund for 1981–1982. After seven months of implementation, the legislative analyst reported that only $22.4 million, or 26 percent of the projected savings, had actually been recovered. The contracting process had become tied up in bureaucratic red tape, partly because it was a pilot project and did not enjoy the full commitment of the legislature and bureaucracy and partly because state bureaucrats held lingering doubts about the efficacy of contracting.[11]

In early 1982 a shifting of political ground began in Sacramento. Legislators and Governor Jerry Brown began to feel intense pressure from all directions to cut programs or raise taxes in order to meet the constitutional requirement to balance the state budget. But 1982 was an election year, and taxes were as popular as herpes. Health and education may have been the biggest programs in the state budget, but it was clearly politically preferable to cut welfare. Welfare reform could save money, and the constituency opposing change was weak; but education reform would cost money, and teachers wielded considerable political clout.

In addition to economic and political forces, ideological forces helped define the legislative alternatives of 1982. Some policy alternatives were more acceptable than others. Legislators had publicly stated that taxes would not be raised, that the budget would be balanced, and that education was politically untouchable. By discarding these alternatives, only health care and the MediCal program remained as targets for legislative change. Two types of changes were considered. California could follow the other states and attempt state-regulated rate review of hospital expenditures, caps on total expenditures, or other regulatory tools applied by the state to the health care system. Or it could try its own version of competition or market reform, which would attempt to change the pressures and incentives to buy and sell health care services.[12]

California ultimately chose its own unique style of policy change and called it MediCal reform. As the director of the MediCal negotiator's office commented, "This was a California phenomenon; a treatment to suit the California disease."[13] This disease, or more prosaically, the political environment, consisted of a long record of defeats for both regulatory and market reform.[14] But the growth of Kaiser-type HMOs, the strength of for-profit hospital chains (some of whom actually welcomed competition), a rapidly increasing supply of physicians, and the new active participation of business coalitions created an ideological climate more favorable to market-style policy change than ever before. The California "disease" was a condition that predisposed the patient favorably to the MediCal policy "treatment" of 1982.[15]

The Political Process

Between January and June 1982, as the Assembly Health Committee staff report stated grandly, "The entire health care delivery system in California, public and private, was transformed from a fragmented cottage industry into a potential state negotiating network."[16] What occurred in those three months was important, not only because of the substance of the changes but also because of the process by which the issues were defined and the legislation was passed. The legislative leadership, lobbyists, and political strategists created and passed two laws that most would have predicted had little chance of survival.

Legislators and Staff

The strategy by which the MediCal legislation was introduced and passed is noteworthy for the intricate way it was steered through the legislature. Every trick in the legislative manual was used; every possible parliamentary angle was brought in to maneuver its passage. Much of the credit for the strategy goes to Speaker of the Assembly Willie Brown (D, San Francisco) and his staff, who had been waiting for several years for the opportunity to introduce this type of reform. Many others, including Senators Garamendi, David Roberti (D, Hollywood), and William Campbell (R, Whittier), contributed as well. Governor Brown, although not involved on a daily basis, was aware of the speaker's strategy and provided his own staff and office resources as needed.

The major strategies for gaining passage of the legislation can be summarized briefly. Business, including the Roberti Coalition and the Chamber of Commerce, was used by legislators to counteract the power of the physician and hospital lobbies.[17] Speaker Brown corralled Assembly Democrats, using the power of the speaker's office to reward and punish his flock. Legislative strategists took highly centralized and secret action, especially in meetings of the Wednesday Group, an elite group of bipartisan legislators, who met weekly for several months to define the direction of the legislation. The usual policy committees, in which most bills are ground up and spit out by the special interests, were bypassed. Four or five bills were introduced simultaneously, with different pieces of reform in each.[18] Substance bills were joined with budget bills, so that a vote against the MediCal changes would have been a vote against the budget itself, a strategy similar to that used at the federal level to pass OBRA in 1981. Conference committee members were chosen specifically to ensure the success of AB 799.

Fourteen legislative staff analysts, who dubbed themselves the "Anointed 14," worked with the Wednesday Group all through the spring to define the legislative alternatives, often meeting in the governor's conference room. Several legislators simultaneously introduced different versions of the policy changes. Some versions were closer to a public utilities model; other versions emphasized competitive contracting by the state. [19]

Key to the legislative strategy was Senator Roberti's development of the legislative cost-containment commission, to the dismay of the Republicans who wanted to claim ownership themselves. [20] Staff to Roberti and Garamendi had concluded that several constituencies interested in health policy change had to be organized and mobilized so they contacted senior groups, labor unions, and employer coalitions throughout the state to find out if they were interested in participating in a statewide organization; the result was the Roberti Coalition. [21]

Business and the Roberti Coalition

Why did the business coalitions agree to become involved in 1982? Cost containment in both the public and private sectors had become an urgent issue for business, primarily because of the cost shifting phenomenon that was affecting labor costs through increased employee health insurance premiums. The less the public payers paid hospitals and physicians, the more the providers charged the private payers. Some estimates placed the cost shifting in California at $0.5 to $1 billion annually and nationwide at $4.8 billion. [22]

Employers throughout the state were feeling the impact of 30 and 40 percent annual increases in health premiums. In fact, in 1981, costs for some health plans were reported to increase from 3 to 4 percent of gross labor costs to 10 to 12 percent in one year. When approached by Senator Roberti's staff in late 1981, key corporate leaders were not only interested in participating but also eager to become involved; the costs of health care had moved business to begin forming business coalitions in California as early as 1978, although most of the twelve coalitions that existed in 1982 were formed between 1980 and 1982. [23]

The Roberti Coalition business members represented twelve business coalitions plus the California Chamber of Commerce. The business membership of the Roberti Coalition was distributed among the following types: 8 percent public entities and transportation, 15 percent high technology, 23 percent manufacturing, 15 percent defense, and 23 percent oil companies. Membership in the ninety-member San Francisco Coalition, not a member of the Roberti Coalition until 1983, was more representative of the internal membership among the twelve coalitions: 14 percent public entities; 9 percent transportation, 9 percent high technology, 32 percent manufacturing, no defense industries, and one or two companies each from utilities, commercial insurers, oil, and banks. No agricultural interests were represented on the Roberti Coalition.[24]

The formation of the Roberti Coalition was accompanied by the usual legislative fanfare for commissions. Press conferences were held, and the meetings were well publicized. Behind the scenes, the Roberti staff had selected their participants carefully to include representatives from the twelve existing business coalitions around the state. Most business members had at least some experience with health care issues because of their experience within local coalitions. As members of the statewide coalition, however, they were generally unprepared for the complexity of the issues and the intensity and sophistication of the provider opposition. "We were hopelessly disorganized and at the mercy of the providers in the beginning," remembers one business member. "They were experts, and we knew so little about the health care system."[25]

The Roberti Coalition met several times in January and February 1982. The physicians were well represented on the coalition by CMA's president. But there were other links between the business and medicine, too. Vice president of Rockwell International George Gamble, the chairman of the Roberti Coalition, was also a consultant to the CMA's committee on health care costs.[26] The other members of the Roberti Coalition were not novices to health care issues. The representatives of organizations such as the Gray Panthers and the AARP had been lobbying at the state and national level for substantial health care reform for several years. The twelve labor representatives included the SEIU, a progressive union in relation to health care benefits.

Although the business representatives on the Roberti Coalition tended to represent large and dominant employers in the state, another organization controlled by big business but with a large proportion of membership from small businesses was gaining momentum in January and February, the California Chamber of Commerce and its newly reorganized health care committee. Although the Chamber had been on record since 1971 in opposition to rate-setting as an approach to health policy change, some individual Chamber members still favored it. In 1982 under the Chamber's direction, Nancy Sullivan, who had previously worked for the California Senate health and welfare committee, set up a workshop for the health committee to reconsider the Chamber's 1971 position on rate setting for hospitals. They did so in March, and on their recommendation the entire Chamber board voted against rate setting at its next meeting. The physicians and the CMA were delighted at the defeat of rate setting but tactically erred in failing to pose any viable alternatives.

The vote against rate setting, along with the providers' failure to pose any viable alternatives, set the stage for the committee to consider other alternatives. If regulation was unacceptable, would the business community support more competitive choices? Sullivan, one of the few outsiders who knew exactly what policy alternatives were being considered in the deliberations of the Wednesday Group,[27] had been in close contact with her former colleagues among the Anointed 14 in Sacramento. She presented some of their ideas to the Chamber, and on April 28 they voted to approve sending a letter to all members of the state legislature recommending the following proposals for changing MediCal : the state should contract with hospitals for services to MediCal recipients; the state responsibility for the MIA program should be eliminated and transferred to the counties for administration and implementation; reimbursement and eligibility for MediCal should be cut further; and copayments should be instituted for all MediCal recipients. The Chamber recommendations were identical to what was then being considered within the Wednesday Group.

It is not entirely clear who influenced whom, but, as they deliberated, the Anointed 14 definitely knew what the business community would support. The budget issues may have created the urgency for action, but Chamber of Commerce support helped define and encourage the competitive direction of the policy change. After the Chamber sent its own letter, they prevailed on the California Manufacturing Association and the California Taxpayers Association to write essentially the same letter to all their legislators.[28]

The Roberti Coalition members, many of whom belonged to these other organizations as well, helped the Chamber lobby the MediCal contracting issue, although the Coalition was still divided with most members favoring a more regulatory approach to policy change. The Coalition had voted on March 23 to support not only rate setting and the hiring of physicians by hospitals but also the MediCal contracting concept. The Coalition's ambivalence about which type of policy change to support partially reflected the diversity of the Coalition membership and the differences between big business, generally favoring regulatory solutions in health care, and smaller businesses, generally preferring decentralized, competitive solutions.

The lobbying and pressure tactics by physician participants on the Coalition did not help resolve the differences either. CMA's proposed strategy for cost containment had evoked anger, ridicule, and hostility from other Coalition members because it put most blame for rising costs on employers and consumer life-styles.[29] The Roberti Coalition members were frustrated with physician unwillingness to produce solutions with real cost saving or structural change potential. They finally included rate setting as a cost-containment alternative because many business members supported the need for strong state regulation to curb the power of physicians and promote effective cost containment in the system as a whole.

The Physicians and the Hospitals

Even though Assembly Speaker Willie Brown had presented his views on the urgency of health care policy change to the CMA in early January 1982, they apparently did not hear him, telling their members in their January 29 newsletter only that "MediCal reimbursement won't be cut after all."[30] By March, however, through their participation in the Roberti Coalition and the Chamber of Commerce subcommittees, the CMA was beginning to be aware that change was possible, although they imagined it would take the form of rate-setting legislation. Even as late as June, their newswletter queried, "What is the MediCal situation? It's anyone's guess."[31] Nevertheless, they identified four major bills pertaining to MediCal and urged opposition of all four, just in case.

The California Hospital Association (CHA) was also represented on the Roberti Coalition, and like the CMA continued to focus on fighting rate setting. The CHA opposed the contracting issues in the MediCal legislation, but its opposition was diluted by a split within the association. Even though the CHA had actually supported a rate-setting model in the early 1970s, all recent efforts by the state to institute regulatory policy change had been successfully blocked by the association, which had turned increasingly antigovernment since 1973.[32] More recently, investor-owned hospitals and some community hospitals had begun to look more favorably on the ideas of competition and contracting. Although the CHA managed to pull two hundred members to Sacramento at one point for an unprecedented "legislative rally" opposing the contracting idea, they still could not agree internally on a unified position. "The CHA saw the bulldozer coming and just went limp," said one member of the Anointed 14.[33] Others disagreed and said the CHA fought as hard as it ever had. Certainly members were active but with a sense of futility. As the vice president of research would say months later, "Change was inevitable, and we couldn't stop it. It was simply the end of an era."[34] It may have been the end of an era, but it was not the end of the story. There was one more group to hear from. One more surprise in the legislative package that would end up becoming the most controversial and perhaps the most far-reaching change.

The Insurers

Early in 1982, the Association of California Life Insurance Companies (ACLIC) held a meeting about the cost shift problem in health care. There was some disagreement within the commercial insurance association about which strategy of cost containment to pursue: regulation or competition. The HIAA had supported regulatory solutions such as budget and rate setting for all third-party payers, public and private, at the state level, and the national leadership generally favored regulatory plans such as those in Maryland, New Jersey, and Connecticut. Some leadership of the ACLIC had always been slightly out of step, supporting a more competitive model of cost containment. The majority of commercial insurers still favored rate setting, but they had begun to despair of ever seeing that goal achieved in California.

At this meeting early in 1982, one of their bright young lawyers suggested, "if you could just knock out the last paragraph of Section 10133 of the Insurance Code . . . that would help us a lot."[35] He was referring to a restriction in the insurance code that prohibited commercial insurers from restricting "freedom of choice of doctors" and "contracting with salaried physicians." This effectively prevented commercial insurers from making any deals for cheaper care, such as those negotiated by the nonprofit Blues in southern California, a legislative prohibition that had favored Blue Cross for years. If these legal changes could be made, then the path would be cleared for changes throughout the health insurance industry, strengthening the bargaining position and market share of the commercial insurers.

The regulation of insurers in California was split between the Department of Insurance, which supervised commercial insurers, and the Department of Corporations, which supervised Blue Shield and prepaid plans. As far back as 1946 the state supreme court had held that Blue Shield was not a "health insurer" but a "medical care organization."[36] These divisions in regulation and law favored Blue Cross and Blue Shield in various ways, and the commercial insurers had been looking for ways to shift the balance to their advantage.

The insurers watched and waited during the spring while the budget process unfolded. When it became clear that the state was seriously considering contracting with hospitals for services to MediCal recipients, the insurers, including Blue Cross, grew anxious about the ominous potential for an even greater cost shift. If hospitals negotiated discounted rates with the state for MediCal recipients, they would most likely increase their rates to private patients even more than they had in the past. Not even Blue Cross, which because of its favored status in the law could ne-gotiate for discounts, would escape the cost shifts resulting from the pro-posed state contracting system. Although Blue Cross knew that changes in the insurance code could give their competitors some advantage, these changes would also greatly expand the negotiating and discounting process in general. The changes would ultimately benefit Blue Cross be-cause of its previous experience and reputation for contracting in south-ern California.

Knowing that their business clients would certainly not be willing to absorb such cost shifts in the form of increased premiums, ACLIC sent a policy statement to the legislature on May 6, indicating their support of contracting for both MediCal and themselves. The policy statement con-cluded that, having reviewed the alternatives, "for now, the focus should be on freeing the public and private health care delivery system from ex-isting restraints."[37] The CHA knew about this policy statement, as in-dicated in their June 2 legislative newsletter. The CMA and the CHA were so focused on the MediCal contracting proposal, however, that they apparently missed the impact that "freeing the system from re-straints" would have on them. Not until July did the alarms begin to sound throughout the provider industry.

The Passage of the Legislation

The nonprovider constituencies represented on the Roberti Coalition were putting considerable pressure on the legislators by the end of April to enact MediCal policy change; the physicians and the hospitals contin-ued to focus on attacking regulation; and a general consensus had been formed between the Republicans and the Democrats of the Wednesday Group that a major restructuring of MediCal would happen.

One example of the bipartisan support that developed for the policy change was the "conversion" of Republican Senator Ken Maddy, said to be a key factor in finally solidifying Republican support for change that the Democratic leadership perceived was crucial. Traditionally a partisan of hospitals and physicians, Maddy gave the provider industry every op-portunity to come up with constructive solutions. He is reported to have said to physicians and hospitals, "You've killed eight proposals since 1977; what do you have to offer instead?" When the hospitals, ignoring his plea, sent out a memo to their constituency, targeting Maddy (along with other legislators) as someone who needed to be "hit up" for their point of view, he hit the ceiling instead and gave his support to con-tracting.[38]

One provision of state contracting with hospitals that the Assembly leadership was pushing depended on a separate office outside the bureaucracy, with a special negotiator or a "czar" as the press later dubbed him. Skeptical of the efficacy of such an approach, the Wednesday Group agreed on April 21 to invite Bill Guy to meet with them because of his experience with contracting as a former president of Blue Cross/ Southern California. On May 5, Bill Guy shared his views with the legislators.[39] Guy's confidence and belief in the contracting approach, as well as his own solid reputation, helped the legislators agree on the special negotiator model and later secured the czar position for Guy. With the Republicans and the business community rallied around, the Wednesday Group was ready to move.[40]

AB 3480 passed the Assembly on May 28, with the czar provision amended back into the bill on the floor of the legislature. From there it went to the conference committee, still without the insurance code changes. During the conference committee negotiations in June, the insurance lobbyists worked behind the scenes to amend their provisions into the law.[41] AB 799 and 3480 were joined together, and when the final vote came on June 21, legislators had to vote for both bills in order to pass the budget. The legislative strategy of secrecy, timing, and power brokering helped the state pass what the newspapers immediately called "landmark legislation" and the California Health Care Revolution.[42]

The Impact of MediCal Reform on Health Care Politics in California

What were the reactions of the various interest groups to the outcome of the legislation? The special interest groups who had lobbied for and against the legislation began to withdraw and reorganize themselves; the health services bureaucracy was in shock; and the politicians were euphoric. The hospital association bravely insisted they had not "lost." One CHA staff member said, "It was not a winner-loser situation." When asked why the legislation had passed, the CHA staff replied that several factors were influential: support by business, commercial insurance groups, and Blue Cross; amendments "opportunistically added" in a strategic way; and prior hospital opposition to rate control in favor of more competitive alternatives.[43] The hospital lobbyists were left to complain only of violations of the "democratic process," a process they had manipulated to their own advantage for years. They later warned their constituent hospitals that unless they bargained their contracts on their own terms they would be "captured and possibly crushed by the state."[44]

The physicians and the CMA had worked hard during the legislative clean-up session to gain back some ground they felt they had lost, although they were remarkably ineffective in changing the final product.

They lobbied in Washington, D.C., and Sacramento and managed to win some time delays and regain some control over peer review and the hospital hiring of physicians. However, they were unable to stop or slow down contracting, the major thrust of the policy change.[45]

During fall and winter 1982–1983, physicians found themselves out of· favor, out of power, and at each others throats. There were exhortations to "communicate" with each other and hospitals to prevent "star wars in the industry." The enemy was defined as "those guys in blue suede shoes [insurers] who may try to practice medicine. . . . Watch out for them."[46]

Given the historic power of the providers, it soon became clear that, if the business community wanted to retain the changes for which it had lobbied, it needed to increase its visibility by educating members about the legislative process. In March 1983, the Santa Clara Manufacturing Group's cost containment subcommittee, held a conference to do just that. The morning sessions were open only to representatives of business and closed to providers. The chairman of the conference received several threatening phone calls from the local medical society about the closed meeting, but the business group held fast. Resolutions were passed in the meeting supporting the legislative gains of 1982. At the same conference, the Chamber of Commerce also released its 1983 legislative priorities: they were almost identical to the Manufacturing Group's. Business had made it clear that regardless of challenges to the legislation by physicians, it would remain united and actively involved in promoting its interests.[47]

The State and Labor

The Department of Health Services and the state health bureaucracy were also affected by the events of 1982. The decision to separate the MediCal czar's office from the bureaucracy and place it in the governor's office concerned many bureaucrats, even the czar himself. "I'm opposed to dividing the administration from the negotiation. It's a lousy way to run government. But if we hadn't done it this way, it would have taken two to three years for the bureaucracy to get negotiation off the ground," said Bill Guy. The state health bureaucracy, therefore, was left to watch from the sidelines as the implementation unfolded, and staff members were forced to wait until the second year of implementation, when the czar was replaced by a commission, to regain some bureaucratic control over the policy process.

The legislators and their staff floated on their sense of accomplishment through fall 1982. Willie Brown's chief of staff, Steve Thompson who had engineered the strategy, commented in November, "This bill has really changed the nature of health care politics. Number one, it has totally fragmented the hospital industry as to how they want to be represented, and the same phenomenon is happening in the CMA. And we've really been able to sell this to the Republicans, this 'free enterprise' model, because it's just capitalism, you know." When asked what the speaker and the governor would continue to support in succeeding legislative sessions, Thompson replied, "We're not going to give up on the push of MediCal into the purchase system of full comprehensive, risk capitation services. That's the policy objective. But we know that the CMA will come back and try to overturn the selective provider provision of insurance contracting. That's the nub of their opposition."[48] Governor Brown, who had not played a public role or exerted strong leadership on the issue, was more than willing to take credit for the legislation once it was clearly a success. At the signing of these bills, the governor declared, "The reforms adopted this year are the boldest changes in the medical industry in fifty years. It finally introduces competition in the marketplace into the world of health care."[49]

Although organized labor did not play the visible role that employers did in lobbying for this legislation, they were actively involved in the Roberti Coalition through unions of retail clerks, steel workers, carpenters, longshoremen, teamsters, teachers, and service employees. Hellan Dowden, the lobbyist for SEIU, commented in spring 1983, "It was noteworthy that anything got through, but I wouldn't call it a revolution. What concerns me are the cuts in MediCal. No one's talking about those, but people are hurting."[50]

The outcome of any particular legislative contest neither indicates the overall power of an interest group nor provides an adequate clue to the underlying causes. For example, the CMA boasted that their political contributions led to the return to office of 90 percent of the legislators they supported and 60 percent of the legislation they endorsed.[51] However, winning 60 percent of the time does not explain whether these wins sustain the core autonomy of the profession or whether major losses might not be followed by major successes that overturn or dilute the impact of the original loss. In spite of legal challenges, heavy lobbying, and new legislation introduced by the CMA between 1983 and 1986 to overturn the 1982 changes, the original legislation remained undiluted. Business and the Roberti Coalition forcefully counterchallenged a CMA bill in 1983, defeating it before it even emerged from committee.

Business

It is clear that business played an important role in the political process that led to the California legislation. If physicians were the "crabs in the bucket" in 1982, then business can be credited with helping to put them there. Business interests in California began to organize to address health care cost issues in the late 1970s. In 1978, Steve Rosinski of Rohr Industries in San Diego formed a coalition of employers to provide support for Senator Garamendi's SB 716, a rate-setting bill.[52] In 1979 the San Diego group helped Los Angeles employers organize a coalition, and in the next several years local coalitions formed around the state, bringing the number to thirteen by 1986.[53]

California was a latecomer to organized business coalition activity when compared to other states, however, This reluctance by the business community to become organizationally involved in health care issues reflects the generally fragmented politics of California itself, the lack of a few large and politically dominant employers such as the auto industry in Michigan, the power of physicians and hospitals to dominate the policy agenda, and the fact that the cost shift had not made a severe impact on California business until the late 1970s.[54]

The formation of the Roberti Coalition in late 1981, as a statewide effort to bring the power of business to bear on the legislative process, was a natural outgrowth of the national business interest in health. The Roberti Coalition strategy, however, was mainly formulated not by corporate groups but by a few Democratic Senate staff and legislators. In forming the statewide coalition, Democratic staff were careful to include not only business groups who were traditional Republican allies but also other organized consumer interests more friendly to Democrats, such as a wide range of labor unions and senior citizens groups. A few provider representatives were also included in 1982; their exclusion would have clearly indicated a loss of power at that time. By 1983, however, provider members were excluded from voting membership in the Roberti Coalition and placed in an "expert task force" instead, an additional indicator of their lost power.

The Roberti Coalition's contribution was not their participation in the legislative process, however. For instance, members rarely testified personally at hearings, leaving that to the more obviously political Chamber of Commerce. Names of individual members were seldom mentioned by newspapers; instead "business" was said to have influenced the legislation.[55] Coalition members did contact legislators privately. Some political contributions were indeed made to appropriate legislators. And the final report of the Coalition did support the contents of MediCal reform as formulated by the Wednesday Group almost to the letter. Business exercised its power instead in more subtle ways, stemming from the structural power of business in society.[56]

The Providers and Insurers

It would be difficult to claim that the dominant provider interests suffered a mortal blow by the passage of this legislation. Physicians were still able to insert compromises that preserved much of their professional autonomy, at least for the moment. But there were several strong indicators that the power of the physicians was weakened by the 1982 legislation:

1. The ability of an interest group to reverse the major thrust of previous legislation in clean-up bills is an important indication of its long-range structural power. In this instance, the CMA was unable to alter the major bills significantly in either the 1982 clean-up legislative sessions or in succeeding years.

2. Physicians did not carry through on threats to mount a legal counterattack through recourse to the courts (their usual strategy) because they did not think they could win.

3. Physician attempts to control the activities and decisions of business coalitions and thus stalemate policy change were largely rebuffed, evidenced by their exclusion from the Manufacturing Group's discussions and the fact that they were dropped as voting members of the Roberti Coalition in 1983.

In the past, individual losses by medical associations were easily overturned, and a refusal to cooperate was enough to produce legislative accommodation. For instance, the AMA's opposition to Medicare in 1965 helped the profession shape the interior of that reform. In California in 1982, the CMA was looking at the wrong interior until it was too late to change strategies; they had already lost substantial power by then.

The hospital association, like the CMA, was considerably fragmented, with some members even supporting contracting by both the state and private insurers. CHA Vice President Bill Abalona later admitted in a news article, "Hospitals are reluctant dragons who must be forced to the wall. Each hospital had so much to lose individually [from contracting], that if the Legislature truly intended to end the cost reimbursement system, it had to act without warning."[57]

If the CHA was able to turn the policy change into an opportunity, so much the better. In fact, although hospitals were to be the main pressure point, they were also potentially the main beneficiary of the new system. The legislation aligned hospitals even more securely, with business and the state against organized medicine. It is not surprising, therefore, that significant elements of the hospital association (including some for-profit hospitals and prepaid clinics) favored the contracting legislation. Other elements, however, opposed it because of economic reasons and the conflict it was sure to engender, knowing too well the limits of administrative control over professional power within the hospital setting.

Hospitals and physicians have been on a collision course all over the country, as more administrative decisions invade the medical arena and more medical decisions become defined as administrative responsibilities.[58] Precisely this potential for conflict, for one crab to eat another, had both the CHA and the CMA stepping gingerly around each other's territory. Certainly one strategy of state legislators was to divide the CHA even further from the CMA and take advantage of the temporary imbalance of interests to strengthen and extend the policy changes of 1982.[59]

A discussion of the alteration of power cannot be complete without mentioning the symbiotic relationship between insurers, hospitals, and physicians. Blue Cross/Blue Shield, an organization started by hospitals and dominated by physicians, had rarely or openly challenged the power of the medical lobbies in California. Historically, the role of private insurance had actually added to the market power of the professions. Paul Starr points out, "The insurance companies used the doctors as gatekeepers to benefits . . . insurance companies' interest in controlling costs strengthened the profession's authority."[60]

In spite of their close relationship with providers, the health insurance industry in California was more diverse and competitive than in other states. The Blues had not dominated the insurance business as they had in the Midwest or the East. Despite their institutional and legal dominance, they had not been a force for policy change in California because of their relatively smaller market share, the intense competition between the Blues and the many commercial insurers in California, and the generally conservative stance Blue Cross had taken toward any policy change.

What caused the generally permissive insurance industry, caught between the CHA and the CMA, to step out on its own in 1982? "Money," as one hospital administrator put it bluntly. The combination of impending cost shifts and a trend toward self-insurance by many corporations moved the insurance industry to action because of potentially lost profits. The new legislation promised some recovery of profits for those companies like Blue Cross that were positioned to quickly take advantage of the new contracting provisions.

Although the insurance companies' support of the legislation was important, it was only part of the support of the business community in general. When asked what role the insurance companies played in the legislative lobbying, MediCal czar Bill Guy did not give them much credit: "The fragmented insurance industry just rode in on the coat-tails. They said, 'Me too.' It was business and the economy that turned the tide."

Discussion

The primary theme of this chapter has been the role of business in altering and fragmenting the dominant interests in the politics of health policy change in California in 1982. What does such temporary dominance suggest for future political relationships? For the health care delivery system itself? Cost control was the major emphasis of business involvement; by that criteria, the California policy changes achieved a measure of success, although business's own employee health premiums did not decline as radically as they hoped.

The participation of business in the 1982 legislation and the continued interest and participation by business coalitions in maintaining the integrity of the original legislation throughout the 1980s is proof that business continues to have a political impact in California. It does not mean that business will replace medicine as the dominant power in health care politics in California, partially because health care is not the highest legislative issue for business associations. The political power of organized medicine was already being eroded by other economic forces, such as increasing corporatization, well before the 1982 legislation. Nevertheless, the introduction of business as a powerful and politically involved purchaser of medical care, along with the state, was bound to change the political equation.

The participation of business alone did not cause these legislative changes to occur in California. But if one combines the power of business coalitions with an economy in recession and a state budget process under severe economic restraint, one can account for most of the political changes that occurred. Macroeconomic forces converged with political opportunity in 1982. The state brought business into the policy process, and the existence of already organized business coalitions combined with interested and knowledgeable state legislators and staff provided the window of opportunity for policy change. No other statewide health policy issue emerged in the 1980s to mobilize the business community quite like MediCal reform had done, but business leaders used their education about health care politics to negotiate deals after 1982 with providers all over the state.

Although the state succeeded in saving money for its MediCal program, it did not put adequate resources into research to monitor implementing MediCal reform. In state government, a cathartic policy change is almost guaranteed to keep that issue off the political agenda for several years. The constituency of the poor is not powerful enough to move issues back onto the agenda once problems are considered solved. As some predicted, "There will literally have to be blood in the streets before policymakers pay attention to MediCal again. That or a decision by hospitals that they prefer rate setting to competition!"[61]

Epilogue

After 1982 the predictions about the impact of the legislation were both unrealistically positive and uncharacteristically dire. The California Medical Assistance Commission (the replacement for the czar) originally predicted savings for the state MediCal program of up to $180 million in fiscal year 1983–1984 and $236 million in 1984–1985, but by the end of 1983 those numbers had to be revised. In August 1984, the state was claiming savings of only $165 million for the first year and $218 million for the second year, still a substantial amount. Of hospitals eligible to submit bids for MediCal contracts, 314 did so, and 246 were awarded; within a year, only 4 hospitals had dropped out of the program, and no hospitals had closed because of contracting. Even the hospitals that did not get contracts had to admire the state's ability to save money. Said one, "If anything good has come out of this program, it's that the state got a handle on MediCal costs. And it's hard to argue with that. The state has a budget too."[62]

The insurers were generally pleased by the results, although the contracting process went neither as quickly nor as smoothly as they had hoped. Predictably, with its experience in contracting, Blue Cross moved quickly to establish "preferred provider organizations" (PPOs) that restricted freedom of choice of physician and hospital for a discounted premium price. By late 1983, Blue Cross had signed up more than 8,500 of the state's 30,000 physicians and 110 of its 500 general care hospitals for its plan. Blue Cross reported interest coming from not only employers but also labor unions.[63] Some commercial insurance companies and even local medical societies formed their own PPOs to compete with Blue Cross, but sales were still reported to be slow in late 1984.

Other consequences of the MediCal legislation were less savory. Within a few years, several research studies began to show that the new MediCal policies might be more costly in terms of delayed care and increased severity of illness than had been anticipated. Christopher Bellavita of Berkeley reported, "The poor, who depend on government for their medical care, are worse off than they were before the changes went into effect."[64] And a careful study done by Dr. Nicole Lurie of UCLA and reported in the *New England Journal of Medicine* in August 1984 found that after six months without MediCal the MIAs whose care had been transferred to the counties had significantly worse health status than a control group. In addition, their perceptions of the availability of care had changed. Fewer MIAs could identify a usual source of care; fewer thought they could obtain care when needed; and fewer were satisfied with their care. The comparison group, unaffected by the legislation, had no significant changes in these perceptions.[65]

Public patients apparently suffered, and so did public hospitals. In spite of predictions that public hospitals would be strengthened by the shifts of MIAs from MediCal responsibility to county health system responsibility, the data did not support that outcome. By the third quarter of 1982, the CHA reported a 91 percent increase statewide in county hospital MIA admissions. County hospitals' bad debt increased by $31 million in the fourth quarter of 1983, and county hospitals had a 29 percent increase in patient days.[66] The California Association of Public Hospitals reported that the nine largest counties lost $138 million from the shift in the first year alone. "Of all the bad debt and charity care in California hospitals, 65 percent of it is now concentrated in county hospitals," said Charlie White of the CHA. "If you want to know the future of county hospitals, there it is."

Private hospitals experienced mixed results from the contracting legislation. Although public hospitals and university hospitals generally had increased utilization, the private hospitals saw sharply decreasing levels of admission. Hospital admissions dropped 39 percent between 1982 and 1984. The decline was steep not only because patients went to county hospitals or delayed care but also because another part of the legislation had defined "medical necessity" even more stringently. So even if a patient needed care and knew where to go, it might be impossible to get that care classified as "necessary." The decline in hospital admissions was attributed largely to the new contracting legislation, although admissions had already started to drop in 1982 because of the general economic recession.

The MediCal legislation clearly had an impact on the California health system. The state saved money, and hospitals costs slowed somewhat to a 9 percent increase in 1984 from double-digit increases in the early 1980s.[67] Patients had a more difficult time getting medical care and thus delayed seeking that care. The severity of illness increased at the same time as unnecessary utilization of hospital services decreased. All these squeezes on the health care system, combined with an oversupply of hospitals and physicians, caused some hospitals to lay off workers, shut down services, and sell their facilities to larger, more stable multi-hospital corporations.

The 1980s began as an era of fiscal constraints, where economic concerns became the new ideology: more emphasis on cost; larger organizations and more mergers; more separation of public from private sources of health care delivery; increasing domination of health policy by corporate interests in health care. When business became an active partner with the state in forming and implementing health policy, some observers applauded the entry of a truly powerful "consumer" interest that would put the crabs in a bucket and keep them there. By the end of the 1980s, the poor and less organized consumer constituencies discovered they needed to monitor carefully the power of this new ally, lest they themselves end up in the bucket.

7

Purchasing Power: Business and Health Policy Change in Massachusetts

IN MASSACHUSETTS IN 1982, health care decision makers faced a situation similar to the one in California. Health care costs were increasing, the state fiscal condition was worsening, and the political process for solving problems was stalemated by provider monopoly over the health policy process. By mobilizing business as a countervailing political power, the state was able to break the stalemate. The legislation that passed in 1982 was called Chapter 372 (S. 2044), a hospital reimbursement bill that changed the incentives for hospitals to provide services and changed the terms of payment to insurers. Chapter 372 was a prospective payment system that used both positive financial incentives incorporated in previous hospital contracts to reward cost-cutting behavior and productivity factors to reduce payments made directly to hospitals.[1]

The compromise that resulted in the Chapter 372 legislation was brokered, not by the legislature itself, as had been done in California, but by an association of large private corporations, the Massachusetts Business Roundtable (MBRT). Through the leadership of this organization, selected stakeholders in Massachusetts health care politics were brought to the negotiating table, and a solution was hammered out in private. The interests participating in the negotiations included the state, represented by Democratic Governor Ed King's staff in the executive branch and its Medicaid program director; hospitals, represented by the Massachusetts Hospital Association (MHA); the insurers, including Blue Cross and the commercial insurers (Life Insurance Association of America, LIAM); physicians, represented by the Massachusetts Medical Society (MMS); and business, represented by MBRT. Representatives of labor and non-business consumers were not included in the 1982 private negotiations.[2]

The role that large employers as purchasers of care played in the passage of Chapter 372 and subsequent legislation was unprecedented in Massachusetts health care politics. The relationship between business and the state of Massachusetts in the formation of health policy during the years that followed provides an interesting study in the fusion of public and private power in the health policy arena.[3] In Massachusetts there was a powerful but highly unstable relationship between public and private interests. By becoming just another interest and participating in the private coalition negotiations led by business in 1982, the state occasionally denied its own legal and political authority and its legitimate role in representing the public interest; consequently public power was not exercised fully. As described by McConnell, delegation of public authority to a private association is characteristic of American political life. The consequence can be a loss of authority for the state, a "permanent debt to the group . . . endowed with authority," and the risk of a "scheme of representation alternative to the machinery of Congress, legislatures, President and Governors . . . a reformulation and redistribution of authority."[4]

In this chapter I will examine the role of business and the state in health policy formation in Massachusetts, the general economic and political context of that policy change, the background of the coalition negotiations that began in spring 1982, the role of business and other coalition interests in the passage of the law, and I will describe the consequences of the business and state alliance on health policy in the state over the next six years.

The Economic and Political Context for Policy Change

What economic conditions in Massachusetts in 1982 created the context for health policy change? Massachusetts suffered the same type of fiscal crisis in 1982 as California and many other states. Although the economic recession of the mid-1970s had been partially ameliorated by the growth of high technology business in Massachusetts, by 1981 high interest rates and other effects of the nationwide recession were apparent in the state. In addition, unemployment had steadily increased from 6.5 percent in September 1981 to 9.6 percent in July 1982. High state business taxes provoked some high technology industries to threaten to leave or move across the border to New Hampshire. The impact of Proposition 2½, a state property tax reduction initiative similar to California's Proposition 13, was beginning to be felt as state money was shifted to bail out burdened cities and towns.[5]

Along with these economic problems, the passage of federal legislation, especially the OBRA of 1981, had the same effect on the Massachusetts Medicaid program as it had on California's. Decreased authorization levels were slated for federal fiscal years 1982, 1983, and 1984. For programs such as that of Massachusetts, which had a growth rate of 157 percent between 1978 and 1982 and which consumed 15.6 percent of total state expenditures by 1982, the federal cuts were projected to be severe in 1982 and the years following. For a state with dwindling budget reserves and a commitment to a fairly generous level of support for Medicaid recipients, 1982 looked to be a bleak year.

Health care consumed almost 12 percent of the gross state product in Massachusetts in 1982, and health care costs were high.[6] In 1980, the state spent $476 per capita on health, more than 41 percent above the national average. Private-sector costs were about 55 percent of total costs in 1980, and public-sector costs were 25 percent higher than the national average for Medicare and 54 percent higher for Medicaid. Hospitals were major employers in Massachusetts, spending 41 percent of the health care dollar, with their costs running 27 percent higher than the national average.[7]

By any standard, it cost more to be sick in Massachusetts than almost anywhere else in the United States. Reasons for high costs included the richness of health care resources (120 hospitals and 3 medical schools, with 2.46 physicians per thousand population), and the fact that these rich resources were overused (the average length of stay in an acute care hospital was 8.7 days compared to a national average that was 15 percent lower in 1982). As long as the economy was expanding and the federal government was willing to pay more to the states each year, the health care industry in Massachusetts prospered. But by 1982, the economy was in recession, and the federal government was not willing to continue supporting health care at past levels of reimbursement.

The participation of business in health care politics in Massachusetts was mainly motivated by issues of economic crisis, high taxes, and high health care costs. The costs of doing business had long been the impetus for business involvement in public policy, and organizations such as the Vault, a group of prominent corporate and banking leaders, had been formed in 1959 to express business interests in social policy.[8] In the late 1970s, some Vault leaders formed the MBRT, an organization that played a key role in the passage of Chapter 372. Although the MBRT had not been organized to address the costs of health care, that issue soon came to the top of its agenda through the educational efforts of state government, national business and some of its own leaders.

Why would business be lured into leaving the secure boundaries of the dark and leathery Algonquin Club for the raucous hearing rooms of the health policy arena? "We couldn't afford not to," said one company executive.[9] The cost of providing health insurance for employees had increased as much as 30 percent in one year, and the profit margins of both manufacturing and high technology industries were in a precarious state. In addition, the political climate under Governor Ed King welcomed business participation, and business had been successfully involved in public policy in the past.

The health care issue most directly affecting business was the issue of cost shifting, whereby each category of payer paid a different amount for a day of hospital care. Hospitals would cover whatever costs were not met by public and private payers (mainly the costs of hospitalizing lower-income and uninsured patients) by charging commercial insurers and other charge-based payers the difference. Because of these cost shifts, employers who insured with commercial companies had higher premiums than those who insured with the nonprofit Blue Cross, which paid "costs," not charges.[10]

Although Blue Cross controlled approximately 75 percent of the nongovernment market in health insurance in 1982, it did not control the same proportion of the market for large corporate purchasers.[11] Of the sixty member companies in the MBRT in 1982, about half insured their employees with Blue Cross and the other half used commercial insurers, such as John Hancock or Prudential. In fact, one-fourth of the Roundtable's board of directors in 1982 were chairmen of commercial insurance firms, a fact that contributed to its readiness to enter the political arena in health care.[12]

The Political Process: The State Brings Business In

Business had become increasingly concerned about health care costs in the late 1970s and early 1980s through the efforts of both local and national business organizations. But to precipitate the political participation of business, it took state action varying from Ed King's encouragement of public-private sector initiatives to direct action by the state's own regulatory agencies.

The state's Rate Setting Commission (RSC), which had authority to set and regulate hospital rates, had increased its already considerable statutory authority in 1978 under the leadership of Peter Hiam, an outspoken advocate of the public interest. A period of suits and countersuits and continual confrontation ensued between the state and the hospitals from 1978 to 1982; business had been involved in neither establishing the RSC nor making its key decisions prior to 1982. Between 1979 and 1980, Hiam and his bureau chiefs decided that the commission needed both a long-term and a short-term strategy.[13] The long-term strategy would be to develop an all-payer system in the state and to involve business as an organized interest group to support that idea. The short-term strategy would be to generate "heat" in the political arena by tightening the system of charge controls on hospitals.

The charge control system was tightened through enforcing existing regulations, until conflict erupted over the proposed changes in Chapter 409 regulations in 1981.[14] Hospitals made attempts to defund the RSC, fire its chair, and change the law. The MHA was mobilized, and Governor King was reported to have received the second largest number of letters ever sent on a single issue when the RSC held its hearing for the new charge control regulations.

Bowing to intense pressure from the hospital association and Blue Cross, Governor King chose to defuse the conflict by persuading the RSC chairman and staff to freeze hospital charges and cap the rate of increases until a study commission (the Joint Legislative and Executive Commission on Hospital Reimbursement) could present recommendations acceptable to all parties. The idea of a study commission as a symbolic defuser of political conflict has had a long history in American politics.[15] The governor hoped that opposition to cost control would die a protracted death due to the boredom of the commission proceedings or perhaps that the hospital association would call off its political attack in exchange for an opportunity to control the process through its market clout, staff resources, and technical expertise.

The RSC viewed the study commission differently. Hiam used the delay caused by creating the commission to implement part of his long-term strategy, developing a constituency in the business community. The RSC bureau chiefs were sent like a SWAT team to the boardrooms of big business in Boston to talk to chief executive officers. Said one RSC staff member, "Business did not want to know that stuff. In boom times, with fixed costs, labor had resisted tampering with any benefits. We went to the CEOs of the mature service companies, the Business Roundtable, New England Life, and the banks. We would just walk into their offices unannounced, and it drove them nuts."[16]

The RSC strategy worked, however, and business became actively involved in the work of the joint commission. One indicator of the change in the business attitude was the position of business seats at the commission table. In the beginning, business representatives sat next to the providers; by the end of the first year, business members had moved to the other side of the table and sat next to state staff.

The Joint Commission and Pressure for Legislative Change

Although a report was filed by the end of the first year of the joint commission, still no substantive consensus emerged among its diverse members about solutions. Unequivocal support for an all-payer system could be found only among the commercial insurers and the rate-setting staff members of the commission. Not even business was fully supportive. However, the commission had accomplished one thing: it had educated the business community more powerfully than Peter Hiam ever could have dreamed. Business had had symbolic membership on previous commissions but had not played an important role except to legitimate decisions and exhibit political consensus. By the end of the joint commission's first year, business members such as Gene Lewis, president of American Optical and a member of the MBRT, could be heard to say, "We're fighting all of Asia as competition; we can't raise our costs more than 3 percent. Why can't hospitals be more productive?"[17] When the business members on the commission proposed a "productivity factor" related to hospital cost control, it prompted one hospital administrator to blurt out, "But there's no such thing as productivity in the hospital industry."[18] That was the point the business community was finally beginning to understand.

Concurrently, the RSC had continued its short-term strategy of generating political heat by denying a contract between Blue Cross and the hospitals, something it had never done before. This denial eventually brought Blue Cross and the hospitals to the bargaining table with the RSC and resulted in a historic hospital payment contract (HA 29), the principles of which were so advantageous for Blue Cross that the commercial insurers wanted them extended to all insurers.[19]

The next stage of political conflict occurred when the HIAA leadership, which was introducing health policy legislation in many states across the country, helped LIAM, the commercial insurers' association in Massachusetts, introduce similar legislation (Senate Bill 495) sponsored by Senate majority leader Dan Foley. Although it was not the first time all-payer legislation had been introduced in Massachusetts, it was the first time the commercial insurers believed their attempts might be successful. The bill proposed to eliminate the cost shift between Blue Cross and the commercial insurers, establish a uniform payment system, and extend the principles of HA 29 to all payers. The bill sparked a fierce and lengthy debate in the legislature, particularly between the insurers and hospitals.[20]

By spring 1982, everyone was feeling the pinch. A new prospective contract was in place between Blue Cross and the hospitals, and the RSC wanted to extend it to all payers. The joint commission was in a stalemate over the all-payer issue, and no one player had yet emerged who could break it. A charge control system under the RSC's authority was looming in the future if the commission failed to come up with a solution. The federal government was readying itself to implement a new system of prospective reimbursement based on DRGs that the hospitals believed would curtail their revenues severely because Medicare represented about 40 percent of their business. The hospitals hoped to escape the DRG system by applying for a Medicare waiver. The MBRT had activated a health care task force and it in turn had been educating and putting pressure on its members who were trustees on hospital boards.

The stalemate was about to be broken. Less than six months after the second term of the joint commission had begun, the commission voted itself out of existence by a one-vote margin. No one can remember exactly which business member cast the determining vote, but a business vote definitely decided it. The symbolic politics of the commission process were no longer viewed by business as adequate to resolve a crisis they perceived as real. Business had fired a shot that, while not heard around the world, would be heard clearly by health policy participants in Massachusetts in years to come.[21]

What or who could take the place of the commission and find a solution to the stalemate? Enter Nelson Gifford, CEO of Dennison Manufacturing Company, vice chairman of the MBRT, chairman of its Health Care Task Force, and political friend of Margaret Heckler (then secretary of the HHS), Governor King, and other influential Massachusetts politicians. Gifford was asked by, among others, David Kinzer, director of the MHA to reorganize the key members of the commission into a private negotiating team that would meet in the conference room of MBRT's offices. Business leaders, hospitals, physicians, commercial insurers, Blue Cross, and some members of the state bureaucracy were asked to participate.

When Gifford took the negotiations out of Boston and back to MBRT offices in suburban Waltham, outside the beltway that rims Boston, it was more than a simple matter of convenience. As one participant remarked, "It was a symbolic move of clear importance to everyone involved." Business intended to use its impact not only on Boston health care politics but on those of the entire state of Massachusetts.[22]

The Coalition and the Passage of Chapter 372

In the two weeks in May between the time the joint commission dissolved and the time the negotiations began at the Roundtable in Waltham, Gifford rounded up those participants he felt were necessary to hammer out a solution and create the coalition. Not everyone who was invited initially wanted to participate. The state was ambivalent. The Medicaid director and the RSC staff perceived a loss of power for public programs in this type of private negotiation. However, the legislators just wanted a solution. Several had walked out of the joint commission meetings in disgust at the lack of progress. They did not care whether Gifford was creating a coalition or a cabal. In order to persuade the reluctant state bureaucrats to become involved, Gifford went to Governor King, who gave his blessing, as did the legislators.[23]

Blue Cross was also reluctant to join. It had everything to gain by a stalemate of the joint commission because it controlled the market and had no particular desire to negotiate away its considerable advantage. Gifford, however, used his status and negotiating skills to force Blue Cross and the insurers to come to the negotiating table and stay there. At one point, Gifford called a meeting with the chairman of John Hancock and the president of Blue Cross. Gifford was in a unique position to broker this arrangement because he was a board member of Hancock and yet his own company insured with Blue Cross. He confronted the two men in the tower of the John Hancock building and told them, "Deal or else." The "or else" implied his potential to turn the Blue Cross board against their president because he had access to at least five of Blue Cross's own board members, who were also Vault and Roundtable members. He also convinced Blue Cross that it had something to gain if it could help rewrite and shape the new legislation, and so it agreed to participate. As its vice president commented later, "We are a creature of our customers and when they ask us to the table to negotiate, we go."[24]

With Blue Cross, the state, and the commercial insurers in line, everyone else came along, even the reluctant hospitals and perpetually recalcitrant physicians. Gifford began a series of a dozen negotiating sessions over about seven weeks. The goal was to have an acceptable piece of hospital cost-containment legislation in the form of a bill by the legislature's recess on July 4, 1982.

It did not happen quite that smoothly. As the negotiations began, each group represented at the table had different goals. The employers wanted cost control and an end to cost shifting through some type of all-payer system. The commercial insurers wanted a smaller and more reasonable differential between Blue Cross and themselves through a discontinued cost shift. Blue Cross wanted both a uniform reimbursement system that the hospitals could not manipulate and the maintenance of their discount. The physicians wanted to participate because they knew that eventually the cost controls would come home to them. The state legislature and bureaucracy wanted to save the Medicaid program money, and Governor King wanted to decrease the power of the RSC. The hospitals wanted to control Medicaid payments so the state could not change the rates every year. Even more critical for the hospitals was a Medicare waiver from DRGs, for which they had recently applied, that was conditional on a legislative solution all parties would support. The hospitals felt particular pressure to participate because business and the commercial insurers were threatening to block the waiver.

Each group in the coalition also had certain resources that Gifford had to take into account in brokering a solution. The employers themselves had the strengths of market and political power, board memberships on powerful financial institutions and hospitals, and the advantage of running the process on their own turf in Waltham. Although they had knowledgeable staff, they lacked the detailed expertise about hospital cost reimbursement and the lobbying and organizational backup and experience of the hospital association and Blue Cross. The commercial insurers had the support of the MBRT, economic and political clout through the power of the John Hancock and Prudential companies, and expert staff support, but the commercials were tainted with a negative reputation of strong self-interest and the economic disadvantage of having a relatively small share of the insurance market. Blue Cross came to the table with all the legal and institutional power it had accumulated for decades, including the contract it had just signed with the hospitals, thus making it "the focal point for regulation of the hospital system." Perhaps Blue Cross's main weaknesses were its reluctance to change its structure and strategy and a public perception that as an arrogant monopoly it needed to be knocked down a few pegs. The physicians, although not particularly powerful participants in the coalition process itself, still held the power of the profession and its perceived lobbying strength in the legislature.[25]

The state of Massachusetts was one of the largest purchasers of health care, both for its own employees and through the Medicaid program; it had institutional and legal authority, a tough RSC and staff who were willing to "play poker" and negotiate. But the state did not speak with one voice and its participation was fragmented by its representatives advocating for differing aspects of state power, turf wars between programs, Governor King who wanted to decrease state involvement and power, and a legislature that had delegated its health policy role to the private sector. The hospitals had never lost a substantial legislative battle over health care cost containment. Their association had a staff of hundreds representing hospitals that were large employers tied to prestigious educational institutions. Increasing health care costs had left hospitals in a vulnerable political position in the early 1980s. Although they could kill legislation, they did not have the power to pass legislation without support. This would be demonstrated forcefully in early August.

How the coalition negotiated consensus is as significant and interesting as what it eventually delivered to the legislature. As the MBRT executive director commented in 1988, "Nelson Gifford wore two hats throughout the process. On the one hand, he was the representative for

the business community. On the other hand, he was the 'honest broker.'"
When the Medicaid director asked Gifford how he could deal with the
complex issues of health policy, Gifford replied, "That's why I'm a broker.
I'm just managing, trying to bring the people together." Gifford knew
when to be tough, when to give in, when to confront, and when to work
one-on-one behind the scenes. Once when Gifford became disgusted
with the coalition negotiations, he told the members, "Look into the pit.
Do you want to be in there? If not, get going, because I have better
things to do. I have a business to run," and then he walked out.[26] Gifford
also used his own board memberships and·urged MBRT members to do
the same. Hospitals began to hear what they called "back pressure" from
their own board members, who were also MBRT members, to go along
with the coalition and find a cost-containment solution.[27]

In public, the Roundtable maintained its reputation as an objective,
educational forum for business concerns. It worked hard to maintain its
image as a "credible, nonfanatic business voice," educating its own members and arguing rationally about health care cost containment. The key
was rational, nonpartisan, issue-oriented discussion. Given the political
context, as long as lobbying or arm twisting was not done on behalf of the
organization, they would not use up its considerable "political capital."

The consensus process that Gifford used was one that was often used
for conflict resolution in business. For the purposes of the coalition, consensus meant that no compromise could be reached as long as any party
objected to it *and* had the power to defeat it. Business was the only interest that could create consensus under those conditions. One staff participant observed, "Gifford perceives of himself as a broker, but he doesn't
perceive of business as an equal player. He thinks business is a buyer
and should control the process. He defines consensus as 'who can stop
this thing.'"[28]

Because the coalition was billed as "just a group of people with similar
interests getting together . . . like you'd have a party at your house," anyone could go home at any time.[29] Sometime in June, the hospitals decided they were not getting what they wanted and walked out. One
participant commented, "It was the traditional mind-set that did them
in when they walked. They had never lost a big one before. The commercials and the Blues were sitting at the table hugging each other for
their own purposes; business and the state were together, and it wasn't
until the hospitals were out that they realized what it would mean for
them."[30]

Gifford believed that the hospitals could not stop the negotiations and
so the most productive work was done during the several weeks the hospitals were out of the coalition. Because there was less confrontation, two
things happened. The bill that the coalition had been working on,

S. 2033, which was a remake of the S. 495, all-payers bill, was introduced at a state house press conference on Friday, June 25. On Monday, as *The Boston Globe* reported it, "David Kinzer held his own press conference to announce that the hospitals would come aboard with two major changes: Medicare had to agree and the productivity factor [then proposed at 10 percent over five years] had to be cut in half." It looked as if compromise might occur after all.[31]

Then it became evident that the hospitals had been negotiating secretly with Senator Atkins to introduce their own version of legislation, an "end run" around the coalition. Gifford got mad. He went up to Beacon Hill, talked to the governor and some key legislators, and decided to ask the legislators to introduce the coalition's bill, S. 2033, for a vote. Around 2:00 a.m. on July 2, they got a reading. "Everyone was there. It looked like 2:00 in the afternoon. The place was filled," remembered one participant. Senator Foley had to concede that he didn't have the votes to get the coalition bill to the floor. But Senator Atkins's bill on behalf of the hospitals did not even get a reading because it was so "fat, so rich . . . it guaranteed no hospital would close." The hospitals tried to play their usual game—"Start with an outrageous position and still get everything you want, but it wasn't working. [Senator] Foley beat them down on a voice vote." While both the coalition and the hospital bills failed to move forward, the hospitals took the harder fall because they failed to stop the coalition process.

It was almost time for the July recess, and still there was no solution. But Gifford was in no hurry because he thought he held the trump card: the power to stop the Medicare waiver that the hospitals wanted. Senator Foley noted in late July, "It's my understanding from talking to many hospital administrators around the state that the waiver is frightfully, frightfully important to them."[32] In fact, the hospitals believed (with very little evidence) that the new federal DRG system would hurt them economically, and they were anxious to obtain the federal waiver. Business, the commercial insurers, and HIAA (their national association) had reason to believe that they could block the waiver in Washington, and they used this threat to get the hospitals to deal again.

The hospitals wanted back in the coalition, but they had to wait to be invited. Gifford did invite them but not until he had assurances both from Senator Foley that the legislature would support a bill if the coalition could put it together by the August session and from the hospital association that they would seriously negotiate on the productivity factor in exchange for business support of the federal waiver.

The next few weeks were a flurry of negotiations. Gifford was said to have spent an entire night drafting what he called the "equal pain" memo for delivery to the coalition the next day. This memo spelled out exactly what was expected of each interest party—what each would have to give. This time when the coalition delivered its bill, S. 2044, the legislature passed it with hardly a word of debate.

On August 10, 1982, S. 2044 or Chapter 372 became law, contingent on the federal approval of the waiver, which was granted by the Health Care Financing Administration in the second week of September 1982. Reportedly, one of the last acts that Governor King performed on the night of the Democratic primary was to get assurances from HHS Secretary Richard Schweiker that the waiver would indeed be granted. The next day Michael Dukakis was the Democratic party's nominee, and King was a lame duck. The new legislation went into effect officially on October 5, 1982. Chapter 372 established a uniform and prospective method of reimbursement for all categories of payers, both public and private, by setting an annual budget for each hospital and guaranteeing revenues to meet that budget, regardless of actual hospital costs.

The Impact of Chapter 372 on Health Care Politics in Massachusetts

As a policy innovation, Chapter 372 was intended to last until 1988. However, by 1985 powerful state and national forces began to modify its scope and direction. The Medicare waiver that was so desirable to hospitals in 1982 was dropped in 1985, and all parties began to consider less regulatory and more price-sensitive solutions to controlling costs. By 1986, when a new commission on health care financing and delivery reform was initiated, the agenda had been broadened to include issues of access and coverage for the medically indigent.

Chapter 372 had different impacts on the various interests after 1982. Business won a permanent and often dominant policy role, along with reduced hospital costs and more moderate increases in health insurance premiums. The state's role became more active through increased legislative interest in health policy and an interventionist governor, and the public share of health care costs moderated. The largest urban hospitals gained an economic advantage, but fragmentation increased within the hospital association. Blue Cross experienced a decline in market share but also had an opportunity to expand into new financing arrangements. Increased cost shifting ended, and market share increased slightly for commercial insurers. The physicians saw a further decline in their access to the policy formation and implementation process, while consumers and labor gained an acknowledged role in the policy process.

The Hospitals

In a memo to members of the MHA shortly after the passage of Chapter 372, Director David Kinzer predicted that Chapter 372 would provide more stability and predictability for hospitals and would keep the commercials from dropping out of the health insurance business in Massachusetts. His predictions were generally accurate, although he underestimated the economic benefits to the hospital industry as a whole.[33]

Data from the state Medicaid office showed that at least twenty-three hospitals made more than $1 million in 1983; this number was up from fifteen hospitals in 1982 and thirteen in 1981. The hospitals that lost money were mainly rural and small community hospitals. In FY 1983, the year after the passage of Chapter 372, the revenues of acute hospitals statewide exceeded expenses by about $90 to $100 million, a 39 percent increase from FY 1982. No hospitals were forced to close.[34] Professor Alan Sager of Boston University has pointed out that Massachusetts hospitals gained from Chapter 372 by holding cost increases at a level lower than the revenues provided by Chapter 372, while at the same time reducing volume, particularly of outpatient and emergency room care. Because of these restrictions, issues of access to care came to the top of the policy agenda by 1985.[35]

By 1986, acute care hospitals had earned more than $60 million aggregate profit since the implementation of Chapter 372. Another consequence of Chapter 372 was further fragmentation of the hospital association, as teaching hospitals and HMOs formed their own associations to promote their differing policy agendas.[36]

Blue Cross and the Commercial Insurers

Section 5 of Chapter 372 mandated a compromise to be worked out between Blue Cross and the commercial insurers through a study commission that would reduce the differential in charges paid between the two groups.[37] The result of both the commission and the negotiations was a compromise in which the commercial insurers gained in political advantage if not in absolute market share. They had forced Blue Cross into a quasi-public negotiating forum to justify its advantage and succeeded in decreasing the differential by several percentage points, from unofficial reports of 12 percent in 1982 to a documented 9 percent by the end of 1983.[38]

Business had insisted that a differential study be mandated in the legislation and that business members be involved. It is unlikely that Blue Cross President David Frost had forgotten about the session he attended with the president of Hancock and Nelson Gifford a few years earlier, even though the official Blue Cross response to the outcome of the differential negotiations was different. A Blue Cross spokesperson commented in 1988, "I would reject any notion that we were under any pressure from our own board to lower our differential independent of any evidence that it was excessive or dysfunctional in any way."[39] Thus, although the commercial insurers gained back a small part of the health insurance market, Blue Cross lost some of its market share as well as its ability to exercise almost monopolistic control over the policy agenda.

Physicians

By their own admission, the physicians and the Massachusetts Medical Society had played a passive role in the passage of Chapter 372. But the leadership of the society knew that physician fees could well be the next target of policy change. In spring 1983, the society commissioned InterStudy to prepare a report on "Chapter 372 and the Physician's Role."[40] The report concluded that by making the hospital the focus for managing the entire health care system, Chapter 372 would eventually erode physician power. The real threats to physician autonomy and authority, however, were no longer located within state or even national legislatures. The threats were more broadly economic and related to the increasing corporatization of medical care and the oversupply of physicians. The new political and economic environment required more flexible and progressive behavior on the part of physicians. By 1987, the growth of HMOs and salaried physicians, the increasing number of hospital alliances, and the ban on balanced billing for Medicare (i.e., Massachusetts was the only state in the country to pass a ban on balanced billing by physicians), all had the effect of decreasing physician power in the state. Chapter 372 began this process.[41]

The State: Executive, Legislative, and Bureaucratic Branches

Chapter 372 and the legislation that followed had differing impacts on various parts of the state. The executive branch gained power through the election of Michael Dukakis, who, to a much greater degree than his predecessor, believed in exercising state power and building and maintaining public-private partnerships and coalitions in which the state could play a stronger role.

The legislature moved from an almost nonexistent role in the 1982 legislation to a slightly more active role by the late 1980s. In late 1987 and early 1988, state senator Patricia McGovern introduced a version of Dukakis's "health care for all" proposal. This was the first state-level legislation in the country to attempt to deal with the problems of the uninsured, and it was not passed easily. The original Dukakis plan had called for a new state health department that would have given the state enormous purchasing power, but that version never made it into the final bill.

The state bureaucracy both prospered and dwindled. The impact of 372 on the RSC was primarily negative. Governor King fired Chairman Peter Hiam in July 1982, during the heat of the Chapter 372 negotiations. All three of its bureau chiefs left state service soon after. The differential study commission gave Blue Cross and the commercial insurers the authority to work out a solution to which the RSC and the hospitals had neither legal recourse nor appeal. And by basing the all-payer system on the Blue Cross-hospital HA 29 contract, the RSC was bypassed almost completely. In the case of inability to come to terms on the next contract, hospitals would bill Blue Cross directly without any discount, and Medicare and Medicaid payments would continue to increase as if HA 29 had been extended.

Some participants argued that the impact on the RSC was not completely negative. "Right now, with compliance, the RSC has more control over the hospital charge book than they ever had," said one staff member in 1984. "It just depends on whether there is the political will to use the power it has . . . with Dukakis in as Governor, a man who won by the use of coalition politics, confrontation is more feared than ever. But you'd be hard pressed to convince me that rate setting is not by its nature confrontational."[42]

By the end of 1987, it was generally agreed that the RSC had, indeed, lost power because of the health policy changes after 1982. New staff and leadership endorsed a strategy of alliance with both private and public interests instead of the former strategy of conflict and confrontation.[43] The policy atmosphere in the state was more accepting of competitive than regulatory solutions. The growth of HMOs and other systems not under regulatory control, the weakening of certificate of need constraints, and the general free market policy ideology promoted by the Reagan administration all contributed to a loss of political power for a regulatory agency such as the RSC.

Other aspects of the state bureaucracy fared better from the consequences of Chapter 372. The impact of 372 on the Medicaid program was quite different from what anyone expected. By a quirk of the formula that estimated what percentage of patient costs Medicaid should pay, Medicaid ended up paying less than anticipated, with a windfall of between $33 and $55 million in unanticipated savings; the former figure is the Medicaid program's estimates, and the latter is from the MHA.[44]

The issue of the Medicaid "double discount," as it was called, erupted publicly in Massachusetts in June 1984. An explanation of the process by which it was resolved can provide additional insight into the impact of

Chapter 372 on the state and the continuing role of business and the coalition in health policy change in Massachusetts. The coalition had continued to meet even after Chapter 372 was passed, and within a few months a bill to correct the double discount was on its agenda. By 1984, the Medicaid "double discount" was the major topic of discussion for the seven-member monthly meetings; a labor representative had been added in 1983 under pressure from Governor Dukakis and Lane Kirkland. Originally the state had not wanted to pay anything back, arguing that, if the hospitals had already charged other payers for that money, then the hospitals would get the double discount if the state reimbursed them. The hospitals then introduced Bill 1402, which the coalition was forced to address. Gifford worked hard with both the hospitals and the state to come to some figure on which both could agree. The hospitals thought there was consensus in early June, but when tested it fell apart. The test of consensus came when the governor, through his assistant secretary of human services, Mark Coven, made public in a newspaper interview what the coalition had been talking about in private: the state's desire to "get something back for giving something back." That "something" was free hospital care for 30,000 general relief recipients as a "condition" of the Medicaid payback.[45]

The alliance between business and the state seemed about to collapse. Coalition members predicted that the Dukakis administration's "going public" might have the proximate result of making the state "an alien part of the coalition" and a longer-range result of ending coalition effectiveness. One participant commented, "If the state is going to use the coalition for its political end before the process is even concluded, without consulting with other parties, then it's not clear we can deal with the state."

At the next meeting of the coalition to deal with the news article and the so-called "consensus solution," the state representatives were *not* invited to the first hour of the coalition meeting—the first time any member who wanted to attend had been deliberately excluded. It was particularly notable that one purchasing sector (private) was excluding the other (public) from the health policy negotiating process.[46]

After an apology from the governor through his coalition representative, the meetings continued. The immediate result was that the coalition held together. As one observer explained the fragmentation within the state team, "The state people would kill to be a part of that club. They won't do anything to jeopardize the coalition process." Another state staff person admitted, "There just aren't any poker players left in the state. They're afraid to confront the other members for fear the coalition will fall apart, but I know it won't. None of them can act on his own any more, not even the hospitals."[47]

Despite this temporary setback for state power in 1985, state members continued to participate in the coalition, and when the next state commission was appointed in 1986 to deal with financing and reform issues the state not only demanded but also won a seat for labor and consumers in general and representatives of the state's departments of elder and consumer affairs.

The Massachusetts Business Roundtable

The consequences for business of the passage of chapter 372 and subsequent legislation were that the growth in health care costs moderated for at least a few years (total hospital costs increased only 6.7 percent in the first year of the system and 6.2 percent in the second, after years of double-digit increases) and business assured itself a place of leadership and dominance at the policy table.[48] Nelson Gifford and the MBRT were perceived as the undisputed leaders of the policy changes of 1982. Every article written in newspapers, magazines, and academic journals mentioned the central role of business in the policy changes.[49]

Would business stay involved once health care costs began to come under control? All participants in the coalition process viewed business as a serious long-term player. As David Kinzer wrote to his constituents in the MHA in 1982, "The most important new thing that emerged from the S. 2044 scenario was the arrival of our Massachusetts business leadership as a 'main player' on our health care scene. They were a new and different kind of adversary with impressive influence and persistence."[50]

The MBRT gave no indication after 1982 that it intended to back out of its leadership role in health policy. Its role in renegotiating the successor to Chapter 372 in 1985 (Chapter 574) as well as Nelson Gifford's role as cochairman (with Phil Johnston, Governor Dukakis's secretary of human services) of the 1986 commission confirmed that fact.

If economic conditions helped propel business into the health policy debate, both economics and politics kept it there. Health care costs did not decrease as much as business leaders had hoped, and once involved in the public policy debate in a leadership role business found rejection of that role could lead to charges of blatant self-interest, contradicting the neutral, brokering role it had tried to promote.

How did business achieve its policy impact? Does the power of business require the type of organized constituency networking that other organizations must use to demonstrate their power in the legislature? During the legislative fight over Chapter 372, one participant commented that the MBRT was not the type of organization geared up to do "floor fighting" in the legislature. If it had come down to hand-to-hand combat on the floor of the Massachusetts legislature, the hospital association might have won. But he also added, "There is a second tier of business power where they're even stronger, and that is board affiliations. And legislators don't want to mess with that kind of power."[51]

Despite fragmentation and conflict within the business community between large and small employers and between manufacturers and high technology companies, despite confusion in overlapping roles of purchaser and hospital trustee, and despite disagreements between MBRT representatives over whether they should play an honest broker or a self-interested role at any given time, the Roundtable remained an effective and relatively united spokesman for large corporate interests throughout the 1980s. Executive Director John Crosier, a former state employee under a previous Democratic administration, helped Nelson Gifford keep the informal coalition active as a parallel force to study commissions and other government mechanisms, and the MBRT increasingly and successfully imitated the lobbying and legislative intervention tools of the hospital and physician associations.

Discussion

Is the participation of business in Massachusetts health care politics and its relationship to the state adequately explained by a pluralist explanation of politics? A pluralist perspective would interpret the events in Massachusetts by saying that business participation was a simple response to rising health care costs. When health care costs increased beyond a certain point, business became alarmed and organized itself politically. It then participated in the policy process more or less equally with other actors, winning some decisions and losing others. All the important interests were represented, and although some interests had more influence on those aspects of the policy process most salient to them, this dominance was temporary and could be reduced by state intervention or coalitions of other interests. The state intervened evenhandedly to assure equal participation and nearly equitable outcomes for all interests.

This perspective, however, does not quite account for all the facts as presented. Not all affected interests were represented, business became dominant in the policy process, and the state was often reduced to the level of merely another interest. Much attention was paid to the statement by business participants that "all the players" were involved in making health policy in Massachusetts in 1982. As I have discussed, however, some major interest groups were not involved at key times. Physicians were absent from the joint commission table in 1981, labor was absent from the 1982 coalition, and organized nonbusiness consumers of medical care were absent from representation until 1986.

In constructing their coalition, Gifford and the Roundtable staff defined "important" and "powerful" as those "organized" groups that had the potential to prevent change from occurring. Clearly, in 1982, labor did not have that type of economic or political power in Massachusetts. Their inclusion in 1984 was not necessarily the result of a more powerful or organized labor constituency but of the leverage of a more liberal Democratic governor (Dukakis) and the pressure of national organized labor.

Nonbusiness consumers were finally included in the policy bargaining process when the governor added a consumer seat to the 1986 study commission on financing and reform and when a consumer member was invited to attend informal coalition meetings in 1986. Consumer representation became politically important because consumer groups had begun to organize and become aware of health policy issues in 1983. By 1986, although they had not been invited to participate in the private negotiations over Chapter 574, there were so many letters to the governor and so much protest over the private policy process that the governor felt it expedient to appoint a consumer representative to the commission on financing and reform.

The consumer representative to the commission, Susan Sherry, was backed by a coalition of groups in the commonwealth that was organized to represent the elderly, the disabled, minorities, women, and children. Two additional state members representing consumer and elder affairs were added to the 1986 commission, although not to the informal coalition that continued to meet. Despite the fact that the consumer representative was an articulate and extremely well-informed spokesperson, consumer interests had to battle for an equal hearing at every turn. Participation turned into power for consumer members when their agenda could be allied with either public or private purchaser interests. For example, the introduction of legislation protecting the uninsured in 1987 was supported and pushed by consumer groups; however, its ultimate passage in 1988 as "health care for all" resulted from the alliance of consumer, business, and state interests.

And what of business participation? Was business just another equal political actor in the legislative game, an honest broker between the other interests? No one involved in the coalition ever believed that, but the process by which the legislation was brokered in 1982 depended on at least a public agreement among all six major players that they were equal at the table and that business was a neutral, objective participant. As one participant remarked, "Gifford thinks business as the buyer can, and should control the process. . . . The risk for him and for business is that someone, probably the state, will figure out Gifford made the public policy process a closed business decision-making process. And it's different. Do we want our health decisions to be made in Waltham and have business shutting the doors on the state when private-sector interests get threatened?"

The decision-making process promoted by Gifford in the coalition was consensus, which was defined as equality of participation and power. In public, the participants accepted those pluralist definitions; in private, they acknowledged a different reality. "All of these people should not have been in bed together," said one participant. "Business was not just 'another party'—it had a definite self-interest in the outcome of these issues," said another, referring in part to the impact of commercial insurers as members of the Roundtable and the conflict that their dual role sometimes produced in the negotiations.

The ability of business to play the broker role and convince others of its impartiality depended on the issue being negotiated. Perhaps if the commercial insurers had been a greater threat to Blue Cross's market share, the conflict between business as purchaser and insurer might have been more aggressively exposed. Or if the coalition had been tackling capital financing, system capacity, or taxation, several participants agreed that the brokering role would have been inappropriate or impossible to sustain either publicly or privately.

Willis Goldbeck, president of the WBGH, believed that business should be dominant in the health policy process. Goldbeck called what happened in Massachusetts the opposite of consensus or participation politics. "Massachusetts was a power grab by half a dozen people. . . . If you have somebody with the pure, raw political muscle to force dominance, you can have everyone around the table, but they're not really around the table. When you enter the policy arena, you are dealing with economic power. And economic power is not played out by hand-holding."[52]

How do we evaluate the power of business in promoting health policy change in Massachusetts? When participants in the coalition would decry business power as mere "smoke and mirrors," a game of power without any substance, it reflected a lack of understanding of the way elite power is organized and demonstrated. Gifford's individual political skills, the participation of multiple interests, and the consensus-building process among the participants gives some credibility to the pluralist explanation of the concrete events. Visible to the participants was the exercise of Gifford's personal power in specific situations, but they failed to observe the way in which power can be understood and demonstrated on two other levels in politics: organizational and societal.[53]

Gifford functioned as the embodiment of personal power, the organizational power of the Roundtable, and the economic power of business, usually the representative of all three. When he put the presidents of

Blue Cross and John Hancock in the same room, Gifford was relying mainly on his personal influence, backed by his own board and organizational affiliations and his status as a wealthy and powerful individual within the community. Within the coalition, Gifford represented the bargaining, employing, and purchasing power of the largest corporations in the state—organizations that represented an economic and political force that could constrain state policy decisions. As a source of economic, class-based power, Gifford represented the ability of large corporations both to identify policy interests widely shared by many corporations and to promote those common interests in the policy process, with or without political participation.[54]

Drawing on the combined power of these three sources, business became a dominant change agent in health policy in Massachusetts. And when business allied with the state's power as purchaser, the potential existed for major structural changes in the way health care was financed and organized in the state. However, there were many obstacles to change. In Massachusetts, business was not always united; Blue Cross controlled a large share of the insurance market; hospitals were also a major economic force; and the state did not fully exercise its own purchasing power.

Although the state allowed private interests to direct and control the policy process in 1982, in the years that preceded and followed the coalition negotiations there was a significant state presence in state health policy formation. Policy making was also a two-way process in Massachusetts: The state initiated the participation of business in the policy process and allowed business to direct and make policy, and the state legislature ratified decisions made by business and its private coalition. Business then organized itself into an entity that, although fragmented and limited in its monopolistic representation of business interests, still managed to put forth its agenda with a powerful effect.

The elements of planning and bargaining in Massachusetts in the 1980s closely resemble Andrew Shonfield's description of French planning in the 1950s: it was "an act of voluntary collusion between senior civil servants and the senior managers of big business. The politicians and the representatives of organized labour were both largely passed by. The conspiracy in the public interest between big business and big officialdom worked, largely because both sides found it convenient."[55]

Epilogue

By mid 1988, events had taken place that raised new questions. Governor and presidential candidate Dukakis's "health care for all" legislation (the Health Security Act) was passed by a 19-to-15 vote in the Massachusetts Senate on April 14, 1988 and signed into law by the governor on April 22, 1988.[56] The bill carried considerable advantages for large teaching hospitals, big business, and the uninsured. The proposal for a new entity that would have allowed the state to exercise its power as a public purchaser of care had been greatly reduced in scope and impact to a department of medical security within the health bureaucracy. Health care costs had begun to rise again in the state, and effective cost-containment options were neither simple nor readily available. More participants were fighting to be heard, and consumer and labor had increased their access to the policy formation process. The strategies of Nelson Gifford and the Roundtable were no longer new or mysterious to the other participants, and business participation at the legislative level had been visibly reduced. In short, the conditions of pluralist politics reigned once more.[57]

Although an alliance between public and private purchasers that could force structural change on the system had not been fully realized, few would claim it was an impossibility. Business had shown it could exercise its purchasing power. Its alliance with the state, while occasionally fragile, still held the power to advance policy initiatives that benefited big business in Massachusetts. Business had answered its own questions about why structural change had not occurred by realizing that small, tinkering steps would not solve the systemic problems behind the spiraling costs. The MBRT executive director concluded, "What we need are structural responses to social issues. Business is the only one who understands the big picture."[58]

8

From East to West: A Comparison of Massachusetts and California

BOTH MASSACHUSETTS AND CALIFORNIA had active business participation in state legislation in 1982, yet the degree of this participation was different and so were the policy outcomes. In Massachusetts where business dominated the policy process, a regulatory policy was passed; in California where business was less unified, a competitive policy was implemented. What economic and political similarities and differences distinguished the two states? What role did the traditional interest groups and political parties play? How important was business participation in each state? How did the differences in business participation affect the policy process? And what can be learned about business participation in California and Massachusetts that could apply to the rest of the country?

Fiscal Crisis and Political Change

The major focuses of political science research on state-level policy in the 1950s and 1960s were state expenditures and their economic and political correlates.[1] These studies concluded what common sense would suggest: that present levels of expenditure are directly and incrementally related to past levels of state expenditure. Conducted in a time of general economic growth, this type of research became less relevant in the late 1960s and 1970s, as many states experienced severe fiscal crises. Political sociologists studying urban and state fiscal crisis in the 1970s began to ask why some states or cities, experiencing fiscal crisis or "strain," had citizen uprising over taxes (e.g., California, with its Proposition 13, and Massachusetts, with its Proposition 2½) and others had little unrest at all.

Why did cities and states cope with political conflict in different ways? Friedland and others suggested that some city and state governments, in times of financial pressure, would develop "reform strategies" to restructure local government, "purge it of obsolete concessions," and turn periods of potential class conflict into periods of a lesser level of managed conflict called "fiscal strain."[2] Clearly, both the fiscal situation and the political structure of the city or state were key variables in producing and promoting these reform strategies.

In the 1980s, particularly between 1981 and 1983, all state governments faced varying degrees of "fiscal crisis" because of recessions, tax base reductions, increased costs of social programs, and federal cutbacks of state monies. In 1982, most states, including California and Massachusetts, had budget revenue balances as a percentage of expenditures of less than 10 percent, and Texas was one of the few states that showed any comfortable budget balance at all.[3]

Following the Friedland argument, one would expect states in economic crisis to form statewide mechanisms to restore the viability of the economic system and provide legitimation for public-private restructuring of health and social service programs. Of all eight states in a University of California, San Francisco, study, only one state, Texas, failed to form some type of public-private cost-containment commission between 1982 and 1984 to address the budget shortfalls and their relationship to health care cost increases. All seven other state commissions had employers as contributing members. Seven of eight states experiencing fiscal crisis did form such commissions and those commissions included the active participation of business. These facts provide a context for reexamining the California and Massachusetts cases. Just how important was the participation of business to the policy outcome, and did the policy solution solve the problem?

Similarities in Economic and Political Context

In 1982 Massachusetts and California were experiencing especially difficult economic pressures, in both the general state economy and their health sectors (see Tables 8.1 and 8.2). Both states had high deficits, relatively high rates of unemployment, generous social programs that placed them within the top ten of the fifty states in terms of their welfare commitments, and Medicaid programs that consumed 15 percent or more of the total state budget.

Both Massachusetts and California had experienced increases in health care costs and increases in insurance premiums well above the

TABLE 8.1   *Comparison of Health Care System: California and Massachusetts—1982*

VARIABLE	CALIFORNIA	MASSACHUSETTS	U.S.
1. Hospital costs:			
per patient day	$510	$548	$430
per patient stay	$3,284	$3,645	$2,486
2. Physicians per 1,000 population	2.17	2.46	1.75
3. Percent for-profit acute care hospitals	30	none	15
4. Medicaid as percentage of total state budget	17	15.6	n/a
5. Health care expenditures as percentage of state budget	29.2	29	42
6. Percentage change of Medicaid per recipient: 1976–1982			
All	37.6	156.8	69.3
Hospital	50.9	88.1	69.5
Drs. fees	43.5	7.9	37.6
S.N.F.	28.2	151.6	55.9
7. Percentage change in Medicaid expenditures: 1978–1982			
All	50.1	66.8	67.0
Hospital	51.4	58.2	49.0
8. HMO enrollment as percentage of total population: 1981–1982			
1981	25	4.0	n/a
1982	30	7.4	n/a

Sources: U.S. Bureau of Census 1982; Institute for Health & Aging, University of California, San Francisco, California, 1982.

national average. Massachusetts had the highest hospital costs per day in the country; in fact, it would be difficult to find a single health care cost measure where Massachusetts was not first or second in the nation. California was slightly better off but not significantly so. Both states had a surplus of hospitals (particularly expensive and prestigious teaching hospitals), hospital beds, and physicians. And in both states, for complex reasons, employers had been paying an annual increase in health insurance premiums for employees averaging 25 percent for the previous two or three years.

The federal cutbacks in health and welfare programs acutely affected all states in 1982, creating a context in which some policy change became more likely. These federal policy changes, accompanied by increasing responsibility given to both state-level policymakers and the private sector, produced a minirevolution in Medicaid programs around the country in 1982 and 1983. All states made some changes in their Medicaid programs, and many states made some drastic changes. The federal cutbacks established a context for change uniting states on the east coast with those on the west coast. Massachusetts anticipated losing up to $10 million in federal money for its Medicaid program in 1982 alone, and California faced losses of up to $40 million.[4] With the new prospective payment system for Medicare, hospitals were sure to face other losses of indeterminate amounts, as they prepared to cope with caps and cutbacks in programs that provided, as in Massachusetts, up to 40 percent of their patient population.

There were political similarities in California and Massachusetts as well. In both states, the executive branch of state government was suffering a decline in power. In Massachusetts, under probusiness, conservative Democratic Governor Ed King in 1982, the state bureaucracies had begun to fight increasingly with each other and the legislature; the once-powerful Rate Setting Commission had been pressured by the governor to back off on the hospital industry; and the joint commission organized to resolve the hospital cost issue had ended in a stalemate. In California, liberal Democratic Governor Jerry Brown had stirred up animosity and opposition from health care providers but had done little to build a constituency to oppose them until 1982. He had been openly scornful of the state health bureaucracy, leaving it in shambles internally, but at the same time he supported a few state legislators and staff in their strategy to seek out private-sector support for public-sector policy change. In both states not the governors but a few state employees and legislators used the fiscal crisis and federal policy changes as a way to put pressure on the provider industry. State employees—rate-setting staff in Massachusetts and legislative staff in California—rounded up and helped to organize business and launched the private sector as a "countervailing force" to industry and other interest group opposition.

TABLE 8.2   *Economic and Political Characteristics of California and Massachusetts—1982*

VARIABLE	CALIFORNIA	MASSACHUSETTS	U.S. STATE AVERAGE
1. Budget balance as percentage of expenditures	0.5	0.1	3.0
2. Unemployment rates			
1982	10.7	9.6	6.0
1983	9.5	6.2	n/a
3. Per capita government expenditures in 1978 (rank of 50 states)	3	7	—
4. Percentage of state in metropolitan areas in 1980	95.3	91.2	75.8
5. Percentage of nonagricultural employment unionized	27.0	24.1	25.2
6. Population density (rank in U.S.)	151.4 persons/ sq. mile (1st)	733.1 persons/ sq. mile (11th)	
7. State corporate income tax rates for business corporations	9.6%	9.5%	

Sources: U.S. Bureau of Census 1982; Institute for Health & Aging, University of California, San Francisco, California, 1982.

Although there were many significant differences between the ways in which business participated in the policy process in each state, business's visible role in passing legislation is an important similarity. In Massachusetts, the Business Roundtable took a leading role in forging a coalition of the interests and presenting a solution to the legislature for ratification. In California, the business community played an important role as well; several business coalitions organized in the state in 1982, but it took state Senate staff to organize a statewide mechanism, the Roberti Coalition, in which business could unify itself and participate. This coalition of business, labor, seniors, and providers gave business a forum through which to express its policy preferences and helped give the legislature the "countervailing force" it needed to pass the 1982 legislation. Although the business community was somewhat divided over what policy direction to promote, the business members were fully supportive of some action in 1982. Their own internal divisions over strategy did not blunt the impact of their participation in the policy process.

Business participation not only shaped the direction of policy change, it also helped shape the process of that change in both states. Legislation is not formulated in public, but in both states the process of conceptualization and debate was even more private than usual. In Massachusetts, the secret negotiations were directed by business; in California, by state legislators. In both states, the usual process of hearings and public discussion was often bypassed and replaced by an alliance between the state, business, and to some degree providers and other interests. The commission form of problem solving failed to produce strong consensus in either state, leading to the private business initiative in Massachusetts and power politics played by the state in California. If the usual legislative process had been followed, it is unlikely that any change would have occurred. Business's preferred mode of operation was much more consistent with behind-the-scenes maneuvering and private consultation.

In summary, both states faced serious state fiscal crisis, high health care costs, and the same federal cutbacks in state health programs. Both states had an active business community available to be mobilized for political action. And both states had dominant Democratic parties and a high degree of political activity and conflict in general. Why did business emerge as a more powerful catalyst for change in Massachusetts than California?

Differences in Economic and Political Context

A few obvious economic differences between the two states might account for the stronger role of business in Massachusetts or the choice of policy solutions. The difference in size between the two states is probably the most salient factor that affected the political process. Size and age of cities have been shown to have an impact on policy innovation in general.[5] Most Massachusetts political activity occurred in the rather small city of Boston, while the California political debate raged the length of the state. The ability of a small number of elites to mobilize and make an impact on policy in a context in which everyone knows the reputation of everyone else is a critical factor explaining the dominance of business. Nelson Gifford and many MBRT members were well-respected and powerful members of the Boston business community. The way in which the MBRT was able to mobilize its members around the health care issue differentiates Massachusetts from California. Although California had a business roundtable, too, it was not central in the policy debate in 1982; instead, California had a "coalition of coalitions" (e.g., twelve regional business and health coalitions), which may have been a predictable outcome of the state's fragmented politics, but it certainly was neither the most effective nor cohesive mechanism for change.

Another explanation for the differences that emerged is the political or policy culture of both states. Massachusetts and California differed sharply in their policy context. For years, public utilities had been regulated in Massachusetts, and hospital costs had been under some type of regulation since 1954. California, on the other hand, was generally anti-regulation. State regulatory control over public utilities had been weak, and proposals to regulate hospital rates or legislate financial disclosure had suffered defeat in the state legislature for more than thirty years.

The Massachusetts political environment was relatively homogeneous and unified compared to that of the fragmented and contentious California, presumably a function of both the size and age of the states. Although Republicans had been dominant in former decades, Democrats controlled the governorship of Massachusetts from 1972 to 1982, and Massachusetts's two U.S. senators were also Democrats. The power of the Democratic party had been increasing slowly since the 1950s, and by 1982 the Democratic party was in full control of the legislature (the "General Court"), a legislature more involved with its traditions than with the crises facing the state. The dominance of the Democrats did not preclude public/private partnerships in social policy in Massachusetts; although Governor King was a Democrat, he was a conservative, and his interests were more closely allied with business than with labor. His Democratic successor, Michael Dukakis, accommodated his approach after his first defeat by King and more actively sought private-sector support for public-sector decisions.

In California, the Democrats had a much more tenuous grip on state politics than in Massachusetts. The Republican Reagan administration ushered in the 1970s and then the Democratic Brown administration reigned for the remainder of the decade. Governor Brown antagonized both old-line Democrats and Republicans. In addition, the Democrats in California did not always vote with their party. Conservative Republican candidates often carried California voters, most dramatically in the 1980 presidential election. California thus was Democratic by voter registration but Republican by voting practices.

California is really almost three states: northern, central, and southern parts of the state have distinct types and styles of political and elite leadership.[6] Northern California is the center of environmental concerns, the logging and wine industries, and is relatively sparsely populated. Central California is the breadbasket of the state, with large and powerful agricultural and ranching elites. Southern California has the highest density of population, including Hispanics and other minorities, and the most industry and housing growth. Southern California also has Hollywood, where politics and theater produced its most famous mutation, Ronald Reagan. California is high tech, huge tractors, and hot new fads, not towering insurance companies, brick banks, and universities.

There were distinct differences in the degree and impact of business participation in the two states. Both states may have had the levels of urbanization, organizational differentiation, and political diversity to foster the development of business coalitions, but the degree of historical continuity and stability of the Massachusetts elite network provided the MBRT with some of the consistency it needed to force change on a reluctant and powerful health care system. The California business coalitions were too fragmented and diffuse in leadership to pull together the business position on health policy change as effectively as they might have. In Massachusetts, one business leader emerged who could broker the policy changes; in California, no single business leader controlled the twelve business members in the Roberti Coalition.

Two major differences in the relationship between business and the state in California and Massachusetts emerge: on the west coast, in a diverse and fragmented political environment, the statewide Roberti Coalition was organized by the state, and thus state interests were strongly represented; predictably, the legislative arm of the state emerged as the policy initiator and implementor. In Massachusetts, the legislature was more of a rubber stamp. The publicly sponsored joint commission dissolved itself, and the private sector coalition, dominated by commercial insurers and business and only marginally representative of state government, formed the legislation and delivered it to the legislature for ratification.

The composition of the business coalitions themselves additionally differentiated the states. In Massachusetts, business participants tended to be large employers, represented by the MBRT. Of its board of directors in 1982 20 percent were commercial insurers, with clear economic stakes in the legislation's outcome. Banks, public utilities, and high technology companies made up the remainder of the board. Small business, as members of the state Chamber of Commerce, was not at all involved in the legislative process. Massachusetts business, at least until 1983, managed to unify the large corporations, high tech companies, and the Chamber of Commerce businesses into a single, rather effective organization, the MBRT, by including associations serving the interests of the latter groups (Associated Industries of Massachusetts, Chamber of Commerce, and High Technology Council) as associate but nonvoting members of the board. By 1983 that rather fragile coalition had crumbled, and the associate members were no longer included on the MBRT.

Business participation in California was less unified than in Massachusetts, had a less concentrated impact on the policy process itself, and represented a different matrix of corporations (see Table 8.3). Each of the California coalitions reflected its own region, but few coalitions had commercial insurers as members, and most included public-sector employers as members. The business composition of the Roberti Coalition reflected the power of corporations from most sectors of California industry except agriculture and insurance. The largest proportion of Roberti Coalition business members came from oil, chemical, and gas companies (23 percent) and general manufacturing and retail sales (23 percent). But 15 percent represented defense manufacturing industries, 15 percent high technology, and 8 percent came from public-sector organizations, a type of organization not represented on the MBRT.

The type of business represented in the various coalitions is related to both the process and content of the subsequent policy changes. In Massachusetts, commercial insurers' prominence as members of the Roundtable provoked charges of conflict of interest. No insurers were members of its health care task force, however, and Gifford disliked even talking about his role as a corporate board director of John Hancock, even though this connection allowed him to force Hancock and Blue Cross to bargain together. The policy consequences enhanced the market position and stability of the commercial insurers in Massachusetts by slightly reducing the charge differential with Blue Cross and by instituting an all-payer system that the commercials favored.

The range of businesses participating in the California legislation also reflected the dominant business interests and the differential impact of health care premium increases on various sectors of business. Large corporate farms in California did not participate. They were less likely to be unionized than large manufacturing firms, and, if the owners were not paying health benefits to their farm workers, they would not be motivated to participate politically. The activity of public employers in the state reflects both the cost of public employee benefits to the state as well as the local history of public-private alliances and the leadership of the state in forming the Roberti Coalition.

The content of the competitive California policy changes offered Cali-

TABLE 8.3 *Types of Business Involved in Coalitions: California and Massachusetts—1982 (in percentages)*

ORGANIZATION	TYPE OF BUSINESS[a]								
	PUB	TRANSP	HI TECH	MFG	DEF	UTIL	CI	OIL	BANKS
Roberti Coalition (*n* = 13 business members)	8	8	15	23	15	—	—	23	—
Mass. Business Roundtable (*n* = 21 boards of directors)	—	—	10	38	—	14	20	—	10

Source: Membership lists of Roberti Coalition and Massachusetts Business Roundtable, 1982.

[a]Pub = public organizations: schools, universities, counties, cities
Transp = transportation industries
Mfg = general manufacturing and retail sales
Def = industries that manufacture primarily for defense
Util = utility companies
CI = commercial insurers
Oil = oil, chemical, and gas production companies
Banks = banks

fornia business the opportunity to initiate various alternative arrangements with insurers and providers to cut costs. The contracting changes would save the state a projected $200 million from its MediCal budget and would open the door for private purchasers to self-contract with hospitals for discounts; this system suited the diverse and fragmented business environment in California. California businesses did not oppose rate setting as a way to stabilize hospital costs, but they knew it would be much more difficult to pass such legislation in the antiregulatory California political environment.

In contrast to the confidence of Massachusetts business interventions, business in California was almost surprised at its own impact. Its leaders were not as well acquainted with the vocabulary or strategy of health politics, but they were well aware of the impact of health care costs on their own profit margins. As business muscle was flexed and the response was favorable, the various regional coalitions grew and prospered. Following the fragmented and diverse California style, no single business organization emerged after the legislation passed when the coalition faced its own precarious future. Instead, local business coalitions organized regionally, chose a representative and a "steering committee" of the three or four California regions, and continued to meet as legislation affected them.

The effect of participating in the Roberti Coalition strengthened the legislative activity of the California business coalitions in the years to follow. New coalitions were formed, and the coalitions united to hire two contract lobbyists in 1986 to fend off challenges by alternative providers such as chiropractors and acupuncturists. The coalitions actively monitored thirty-three bills in 1988 and sponsored a data bill to force greater disclosure of health care information to employers.[7]

What about the way health care politics was played in both states? In Massachusetts, the most powerful institutional forces were Blue Cross and the hospitals. Blue Cross dominated the Massachusetts insurance market, but the commercial insurers had the power associated with their alliance with business through the MBRT. In California, Blue Cross had to fight with dozens of active commercial insurance plans plus a popular and established HMO movement. Physicians on both coasts were still powerful but suffering internal divisiveness and fragmentation due to oversupply and overconfidence. Massachusetts acute care hospitals were either community nonprofit or teaching nonprofit, and they were very successful as a political lobbying force.[8] Although the hospitals were divided between teaching hospitals and community hospitals, the hospital association could still exert considerable power in the legislature to block change. Hospitals in California were more evenly divided between for-profit, nonprofit, public hospitals, HMO hospitals, and clinics. The division resulted in their inability to unite behind a single position and oppose the 1982 legislation with the force and success they had had in earlier years.The differences between the two states in the early 1980s point to a contrast between Massachusetts, a stable, homogenous state with well-organized elites but a relatively weak legislative branch, and California, a fragmented, volatile state with decentralized power centers, little historical continuity between the business elites involved in health care politics, and an active legislative branch. Massachusetts gained a stronger executive branch and an even more interventionist state with the election of Governor Michael Dukakis in 1982, while California lost considerable intervention potential with the election of Republican Governor George Deukmejian the same year. Thus, the strength of business in Massachusetts health care politics was associated with increased state presence in the years to follow, while the fragmentation of business in California was accompanied by the increased fragmentation of other interests, including the state. The political consequences of these different environments are identifiable in the policies that resulted from those changes.

Similarities and Differences in Policy Outcomes

The policy consequences in both states were legislative changes that defused conflict and postponed both state and private-sector fiscal crisis in the health sector. The political outcome in both states was a strengthened business presence in health care politics and, in combination with other forces of increasing corporatization in health care, a weakening of traditional organized forces, such as insurers, hospitals, and physicians. When purchasers and the state ally to force change on providers, a realignment of political forces can occur.

It has been claimed that California, a politically conservative state, put forth a radical solution for two levels of care, while Massachusetts, a liberal state, proposed a conservative solution with a single standard of care. The evidence does not support those labels. The 1982 California legislation led the way to an even more pronounced multitiered system of care. By 1984 the evidence was beginning to suggest that the poor had been further fractioned into MediCal poor and MIA poor.[9] The transfer of MIAs from state to county responsibility with a decrease in funding raised other kinds of questions in California about whether MIAs were "medical care dropouts" or whether MIAs were delaying necessary care until their conditions became urgent. State contracting with the private sector or private-sector contracting with other private entities could hardly be considered "radical," given that it is an ordinary process for all types of government and private services.

In California only a few hospitals closed in the following years, and it is unlikely that MediCal reform alone was the culprit. Although fewer PPOs were being formed by 1984 than expected, by 1986, PPO activity had begun to increase again in the state. And although hospitals initially opposed the legislation, they were actively contracting by 1983 with both the state and major employers. Physicians were being polarized into those who did and those did not—sign up with PPOs or HMOs, that is.

HMO enrollment almost doubled in Massachusetts in the year following its regulatory solution, while enrollment in "competitive" California increased only slightly. Massachusetts, on the other hand, touted its legislation as having a social orientation and maintaining a single standard of care. Underneath the veneer of a single standard, however, its Medicaid recipients had the same problem gaining access to providers as in California, and, after the 1982 legislation, there were widely reported efforts to dump public patients from private into public hospitals. MIAs did not have any inpatient hospital coverage at all in Massachusetts, leading to the "free care flap" of the Dukakis administration in 1984 and a commission to address the needs of the medically indigent and uninsured in 1986.[10] The Massachusetts solution was relatively conservative, considering the maintenance of power for organized interests. Teaching hospitals were preserved, although some smaller community hospitals were beginning to face financial difficulties in the late 1980s.

The differences between Massachusetts and California were not so dramatic as they were portrayed at the outset by the press and the participants. Kinzer said, "It is hard to imagine how the divergent approaches taken by California and Massachusetts will ever be reconciled. . . . It seems unlikely that the result will be something in between." He apparently had not heard about Florida or Wisconsin, where the results were a mixture of regulation and competition, nor did he take into account the pragmatism of business or the compelling reasons for alliances between business and the state.[11]

Discussion

The emergence of organized business interests in alliance with the state provided an opportunity for the state to tip the distributive balance away from dominant provider or producer interests and toward purchaser (state and business) interests in both Massachusetts and California. Once aware in a collective way of how they could benefit from political participation, the business representatives in both states participated vigorously. In Massachusetts, the political and economic interests of the state and the financial interests of the commercial insurers declared a fiscal emergency and prodded the large corporate interests to get politically involved. Certainly both states faced urgent pressure to balance their budgets. The cases have provided ample data to support that urgency and its definition as beyond the control of any one state sector. The policy changes that the business sectors promoted were aimed at increasing public-sector productivity. To the extent that hospital and health care costs stabilized or decreased, the policy changes (along with other economic factors) were successful in reducing the fiscal crisis at the state level.

In both states, fiscal crisis produced the context in which policy change was possible. In neither state was the proposed policy change new. Both states had introduced similar legislation in previous years, laying the groundwork for what was perceived as dramatic or revolutionary changes in 1982. Although business was already organized in both states, state staff and leadership brought business into the public policy debate. Once involved, business power was dominant in the Massachusetts policy process but less so in California. Factors of political culture, fragmentation, and size of the state all contributed to the relatively less powerful role of business in California. The policy changes that resulted from the business-state alliances in Massachusetts and California resulted in a more powerful private sector in both states.

The questions raised by this discussion lead the observer to consider California and Massachusetts in the context of fifty-state business activity and health policy change as described in the next chapter. How can the experiences of these two states be placed into the context of activity in all fifty states? To what degree is strong business participation associated with certain types of policy change?

9

Business in the Fifty States

MASSACHUSETTS AND CALIFORNIA are extreme states—coastally sophisticated, urban, innovative. Business might have been active in these places, but what about Iowa, Arizona, and Tennessee? How active was business in the fifty states, and what types of policy change did business support or oppose? This chapter will describe the policy menu in the early 1980s and the choices business made, the varying levels of business participation around the country, and the way business participated in two types of health policy change that were highly controversial—financial disclosure of health care costs and state rate regulation of hospital costs. The data presented here will not describe whether the participation of business caused these policy changes to occur at the state level. Too many other factors would have to be included to make such a connection (that is, levels of urbanization, unionization, costs of medical care, degrees of state fiscal crisis, etc.). However, one can learn something about how extensive business intervention was and whether business supported any patterns of policy change at the height of business interest in the mid-1980s.

The Health Policy Menu in the 1980s

As business representatives struggled over effective approaches to health care cost containment, they were operating within a context of a profound paradigm shift in the health policy debate between the mid-1960s and the mid-1980s. At least four types of shift in thought influenced the policy alternatives available for discussion and implementation: (1) shifts from an emphasis on access in the mid-1960s to the cost of medical care by the mid-1980s;[1] (2) ideological shifts from regulatory to market approaches to policy change;[2] (3) shifts in the role of government from provider and passive financer to more aggressive purchaser;[3] and (4) shifts in the location of decision making and accountability from the federal to the state level.[4] I have provided evidence of these shifts in previous chapters in the way business became involved in cost containment in the 1970s, the way the Reagan administration molded the policy debate and emphasized market reform as well as state responsibility, and the increased degree and intensity of health policy activity at state and local levels all around the country in the early 1980s.

Health policy alternatives were discussed in the "either-or" nature of the competition-regulation debate throughout the 1980s.[5] As Democrats struggled to become as market-oriented as the Republicans, some Republicans turned to supporting the regulation of health care as a cost-containment strategy. The rhetoric of the debate created an atmosphere in which definitions either were not made at all or when they were they obscured the underlying arguments about health policy change.[6]

Although the market strategies were sometimes difficult to identify, policymakers seemed to know a regulatory solution when they saw one. For David Winston, President Reagan's White House czar, "statewide efforts to control health care costs" were equivalent to state rate setting and thus regulation. For others, regulatory strategies were synonymous with "command and control," "federal intervention," "health planning," and even "socialism." Given various regulatory strategies, some centralized and others decentralized, the issue became further complicated. The key words that seemed to distinguish regulation from competition in the minds of the devoted of either persuasion were "mandate" (or "impose") and "foster." If the federal government repealed or modified a law, as it did in 1981 and 1982 with regard to HMO regulations and Medicaid requirements, with the intent of removing artificial barriers to free competition in the marketplace, then the change fostered competition. If the government set a cap on reimbursement or mandated certificate of need programs, the change was mandatory and thus regulatory. In both cases, the source of change was centralized with the federal government. As Daniel Sigelman has suggested, "Beneath surface hostility to regulation, however, lies a system that creates and depends on perhaps even more regulation than current exists. . . . A vast web of federal regulation has been aimed directly at providers . . . under the competitive approach."[7]

In the 1980s business variously supported or opposed two types of policy change in the fifty states: state or federal financial disclosure of health care costs and hospital all-payers rate setting. State rate-setting or rate review of hospital charges is the most common policy alternative generally agreed to be regulatory in nature. The regulation of public utilities at the state level has a history of almost one hundred years in the United States. State rate regulation in the hospital industry is more recent, beginning seriously in the early 1970s. The control of hospital costs was and remains the target of this cost-containment strategy because hospital spending has consistently accounted for nearly half of all personal health care expenditures. Hospital price controls or state rate-setting programs have been the most controversial of the efforts to control hospital expenditures. Mandatory control programs, in which all general acute care hospitals must comply with state rate-setting regulations and where the authority to force compliance rests with a government agency or commission, were found in nine states (i.e., Massachusetts, Connecticut, New York, Maryland, Washington, Wisconsin, New Jersey, Maine, and West Virginia) for all payers (public and private) by the end of 1984; in eight more states (i.e., Rhode Island, Oregon, Indiana, Florida, Arizona, Alaska, Virginia, and Vermont) the form of rate setting for some payers or voluntary rate review was established; and additional legislation to regulate hospital costs was introduced in eight states (Arizona, Florida, Illinois, Indiana, Kansas, Utah, Vermont and Wyoming) in 1984. In 1984 this left only thirteen states around the country in 1984 that did not already have rate setting or review or were not seriously considering and discussing it.[8]

One major reason why business would support a regulatory policy such as rate setting is that it can offer some cost savings by reducing the rate of growth in hospital costs by as much as four percent a year.[9] The fact that these reductions have traditionally been associated with the eastern states where the population may be older and sicker than in other areas suggests that the cost savings might be even greater if case mix were taken into account. Business also supports all-payer rate setting because it prevents cost shifts from the public sector to the private sector. When the public sector becomes an aggressive purchaser and clamps down on its costs, as it has in the past twenty years for Medicare and Medicaid, hospitals have traditionally shifted those costs to the private payer. These cost shifts to the private sector helped propel business into the health policy debate in the first place.

The market strategies are much more varied and difficult to define. As Lawrence Brown has observed, "Market reform proposals require the federal government to design with care and specificity a set of top-down rewards and penalties which, when applied to the system from above, may be depended on to change millions of individual choices significantly in directions that government prefers and that the individuals affected hitherto rejected."[10] As proposed by the Reagan administration in the 1980s, the procompetition or market strategies included the establishment of competing alternative health plans such as HMOs or PPOs, tax reform proposals to tax either employee or employer contributions to health benefit plans, and the disclosure of price and quality information about health care to make consumers and purchasers better informed buyers.

The most successful of the federal market strategies was the passage of the prospective payment system in 1983 in which the government paid a fixed amount to hospitals for Medicare beneficiaries for the treatment of specific disease categories. But PPS was not particularly competitive because government set the categories that it would reimburse and the limit for that reimbursement. Hospitals were left to shift costs to the private charge payers or encourage admissions or whatever else they needed to do to keep within the budgetary limits. By the end of the 1980s, there was evidence that while hospital length of stay had declined, hospital costs still continued to increase.[11]

Where has business been in the regulation-competition debate? The leaders of business have not been fooled by the false dichotomies between regulatory and competitive strategies for cost containment. As Paul Ellwood comments, "Business support for government regulation has been jarring. In the tug of war between government regulation and market forces, business leaders have traditionally sided with the market. . . . Why, then have employers adopted an uncharacteristic regulatory stance in health care matters? Simply because they are frustrated. Although they like the theory behind the market approach, it has not worked quickly enough for them."[12] Willis Goldbeck of the Washington Business Group on Health agrees, "Sure the rhetoric of business supports competition, but the rhetoric means nothing. Business has never been in favor of competition. They want to regulate everything as long as it's not them. This $400 billion issue will not be played out on the basis of rhetoric."[13]

While the rhetoric and ideology of competition may be favored and supported by small business, big business has tended to support both regulatory and market policy solutions. The interests of big business have been to contain costs, rationalize the system, and discipline physicians, not to get enmeshed in the rhetoric of the policy debate. Whatever works and whatever produces change most quickly has been the position of most larger business organizations. It has not been a question of whether to regulate, but what type of regulation and at what level.[14] When costs were at their highest in the early 1980s, business representatives were involved in various strategies at the local and state level, both regulatory and competitive.

Levels of Business Participation

It is fairly clear that business was active in California and Massachusetts in the early 1980s, but how can one characterize such activity on a broader scale? Asking people what they think about business participation requires that their biases be taken into account. Counting the number of coalitions around the country means assuming that the more coalitions there are, the more active business will be.

In order to classify and characterize levels of business participation in the various states, I chose to combine measures from three fifty-state telephone surveys conducted in late 1983 and early 1984: the Federation of American Hospitals,(FAH) survey of fifty state hospital associations; a Chamber of Commerce of the U.S. annual survey of business coalitions, published in the Chamber's 1984 "Directory of Business Coalitions for Health Action"; and a fifty-state survey of state rate regulation and business activity conducted by InterStudy in November 1983.[15] I chose to focus on the period between 1982 and 1984 for two reasons: it coincided with the time period covered by the two state case studies, and it represented the period of the highest degree of business coalition activity around the country as measured by the number of new coalitions being formed between 1982 and 1984.[16] If I could capture a snapshot of business activity in the fifty states during what everyone admits was its highest point, it would be easier to compare earlier or later levels of intervention in relationship to the peak of participation.

By combining the responses to these three surveys, I constructed categories of business participation that included two sets of perceptions of business activity (both from surveys of hospital association representatives) and one more objective measure, the actual number of business coalitions in a given state. Certainly I do not consider hospital association representatives the last or even latest word on business coalition activity; however, I felt that the tendency by some representatives to exaggerate the power of business coalitions would probably be offset by the tendency of others to play it down. By including a measure of the actual number of coalitions, I hoped to obtain a composite measure that would be a more valid estimate of business participation around the country. Because both surveys explicitly asked about health policy changes at the state level in late 1983 and early 1984 and attempted to link those changes to business coalition activity, I had two unrelated sources of information that I could correlate with other sources about health policy change at the state level.

The Federation of American Hospitals Survey

The FAH survey asked state hospital association representatives to characterize the level and intensity of business activity related to health policy changes in their states. The survey also asked ten other questions about specific health policy changes during 1984, such as the passage of financial disclosure laws, rate-setting programs, Medicaid program changes, and prospects for legislative change in 1985. All fifty state hospital associations responded to the survey. The survey asked each hospital asociation representative, "Is there business activity under way in your state? If so, what is its level and intensity?"

All fifty states made some type of response to the business coalition question. Only two states—West Virginia and South Dakota—responded with a single word answer, "none." All other responses contained at least one sentence of description about the type and level of business activity. Eighteen states reported a high degree of interest and/or participation by business groups in more than one area of the state; I labeled these states "high business participation" states. Seventeen states reported some interest or participation, usually beginning activity in one area of the state; I labeled these states "medium business participation" states. And fifteen states reported minimal interest or no activity at all; I called these states "low business participation" states. For the definition of "business participation," I used the FAH respondents' own terms, although they often did not distinguish between participation, interest, and activity.

The U.S. Chamber of Commerce Survey

The Chamber of Commerce of the U.S. survey of coalitions in 1984 attempted to compile the most complete information possible on the status and activities of the 146 coalitions that were in various stages of development by early 1984. The national Chamber staff made inquiries by telephone and mail to all local Chambers of Commerce and to coalitions that had responded to earlier surveys. By the end of 1983 forty-three states, including the District of Columbia, reported at least one business/health coalition to the Chamber.[17] Combining the data from both the FAH survey and the Chamber of Commerce directory, I concluded that at least forty-three and perhaps as many as forty-six states had at least one business and health coalition by 1984.[18]

Using the Chamber reports on numbers of coalitions in each state, I grouped the states into the same three categories as the FAH survey: low business participation = states with no report or only one coalition; medium business participation = states with two or three coalitions; and high business participation = states with five or more coalitions.[19] The

FAH and Chamber data placed thirty-one states into the same category. Because there were discrepancies for nineteen states, the InterStudy survey became useful.

The InterStudy Survey

In late 1983, about the same time that the Chamber was collecting its data from business coalitions, InterStudy, a policy research institute in Minnesota, did a telephone interview survey with fifty state hospital associations to determine the status of hospital rate regulation in the fifty states and the role business had played in promoting or opposing all-payer systems. Although the reports of business activity were specifically related to the role of business over one policy issue, it seemed plausible that in states where business had been active, either for or against rate setting, there might be a high degree of business participation in other health policy issues. In order to support or oppose rate setting, a business representative or organization would have to be knowledgeable about health care cost containment.

Because I had two measures of business activity and some discrepancy over how to categorize nineteen states, I used the InterStudy report to help resolve the differences and assign a final category of business participation. States were assigned to a category if two out of the three reports agreed on the level of participation. Only three states had no agreement among the three surveys, and these states—Texas, Minnesota, and Kentucky—were assigned to a medium category. (See Appendix A for a list of all fifty states and their levels of participation as defined by all three surveys.) Table 9.1 and Figure 9.1 show all fifty states and their levels of participation. Using the combined measure of levels of participation sixteen states fell into the low business participation category; sixteen in the medium category; and eighteen in the high category. There was a surprising consistency between the three surveys in the final grouping, with complete agreement between the three surveys for almost half the states (twenty-one) and only one category difference for an additional twenty-two states. These groupings are not meant to be definitive, but they simply suggest one way of looking at levels of business participation in the fifty states in the mid-1980s.

Business and Health Policy Change in the Fifty States: The Case of Financial Disclosure and Rate Setting

Using data available from the FAH and InterStudy surveys of health policy change in the fifty states, I selected two types of policy change

TABLE 9.1   *Combined Measure of Business Participation in the Fifty States*

Group 1: Low Business Participation (16 states)

Alaska	Mississippi	New Mexico
Arkansas	Montana	North Dakota
Idaho	Nebraska	Rhode Island
Louisiana	Nevada	South Dakota
Maine	New Hampshire	West Virginia
		Wyoming

Group 2: Medium Business Participation (16 states)

Alabama	Kentucky	Texas
Colorado	Maryland	Utah
Delaware	Minnesota	Vermont
Georgia	New Jersey	Virginia
Hawaii	Oregon	Washington
		Wisconsin

Group 3: High Business Participation (18 states)

Arizona	Iowa	North Carolina
California	Kansas	Ohio
Connecticut	Massachusetts	Oklahoma
Florida	Michigan	Pennsylvania
Illinois	Missouri	South Carolina
Indiana	New York	Tennessee

Sources: U.S. Chamber of Commerce Survey 1984; InterStudy Survey 1983; FAH Survey 1984.

with which to associate levels of business participation: the existence of and pressure for financial disclosure and rate-setting laws at the state level. The quest for information about health care costs has been one of the first priorities of every business coalition. However, procuring data often requires state legislation and a strong political challenge to existing provider interests by employers and their associations. What role has business played throughout the country in promoting the passage of such legislation?

The FAH survey asked hospital representatives, "Are hospitals in your state feeling pressure from legislators, business coalitions, or others for financial disclosure or comparison of charges?" In most states, the an-

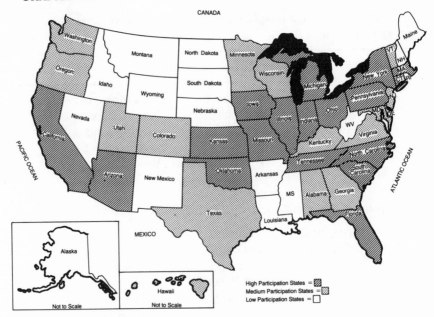

FIG. 9.1

swers were descriptive beyond a simple yes or no, allowing the answers to be coded into three categories: "Yes"—states had some type of mandatory financial disclosure law; "Some"—states where financial disclosure was being discussed or there was specific pressure for disclosure; "No"—states that had no disclosure or no pressure for disclosure. Nineteen states reported that they already had some type of mandatory financial disclosure; nineteen states reported pressure from various sources; and twelve states reported no activity.[20]

As I demonstrate in Table 9.2, 56 percent of the states in which business participation was classified as high had financial disclosure laws in contrast to only 13 percent of the low participation states. Conversely, of the low participation states, 50 percent reported no financial disclosure laws while only 11 percent of the high states were without this legislation (see Appendix B for a list of the states in each cell). The differences between the two groups were clear and strong, as the measures of association in the table indicate. States in which business participation was high had laws guaranteeing the right of access by employers and other groups to hospital and/or physician cost data through the passage of financial disclosure legislation. Of the low participation states, not a single state respondent to the survey mentioned any pressure from business coalitions for financial disclosure. Of the medium participation states, there were specific references to business pressure in 19 percent of the state re-

TABLE 9.2   *Existence of Financial Disclosure Laws in 50 States by Levels of Business Participation, 1984 (in percentages)*

FINANCIAL DISCLOSURE	HIGH BUSINESS	MED. BUSINESS	LOW BUSINESS	TOTAL
None[a]	11 (2)	12 (2)	50 (8)	24 (12)
Some[b]	33 (6)	44 (7)	37 (6)	38 (19)
Yes[c]	56 (10)	44 (7)	13 (2)	38 (19)
Totals	100 (18)	100 (16)	100 (16)	100 (50)

Sources: Data use the combined measure of business participation for the independent variable. For the dependent policy variables, see data from Cyndee Eyster, "Special Report on Health Issues in Election Year '84: State Roundup," *Review* 17:5 (September/October 1984):16–35; and Barbara Paul, "State-by-State Hospital Rate Regulation Survey: Movement Toward All-Payers System and the Role of Business in Promoting All-Payers Systems," Memorandum (Excelsior, Minn.: InterStudy, 4 November 1983): 1–26.

Note: Measures of association are Chi square = 11.21
Effect parameter = + 21
[a]None = No financial disclosure laws existed in the state.
[b]Some = Voluntary disclosure existed or laws were being discussed.
[c]Yes = Financial disclosure laws existed and were mandatory for all hospitals.

sponses. Of the high participation states, 61 percent made a specific reference to business participation or pressure.[21]

Although I cannot prove by these data alone that business caused the passage of these laws, there is definitely a strong association between the existence of business activity and the existence of these laws. The fact that most business coalitions were formed in the year or two prior to the passage of these laws in most states, and that the Washington Business Group on Health had made financial disclosure one of its top priorities in 1982, lends strength to the plausibility of a causal connection. Furthermore, the financial disclosure issue began at the state level, where business influence was strongest in the early 1980s.

The relationship of business participation to the regulation of health care costs is not clear. Within states and within business coalitions there has been considerable debate over the efficacy and appropriateness of rate setting as a policy solution. As I observed in the California case, business was divided over whether to support rate setting in the state in 1982, eventually choosing what seemed to be the most pragmatic and workable solution for change. In Massachusetts, because of its regulatory history, the participation of big business, and the disposition of the commercial insurers toward regulation, a rate-setting solution for all payers was more readily acceptable to the business participants.

Table 9.3, based on data from both the FAH and the InterStudy survey, shows, not surprisingly, that there was essentially *no* detectable relationship between the level of business participation and the existence of state rate-setting programs. (The effect parameter is essentially zero, and the chi-square is very low.) The table divides rate-setting programs into three categories: Yes—states where there was mandatory rate setting in 1984; Some—states where there was voluntary rate review, serious discussion about the introduction of rate-setting legislation, or recent defeats for rate setting; and No—states where there was essentially no interest in rate setting and no legislation being introduced to deal with it. (See appendix C for a list of the states in each cell of Table 9.3.) The same number of high business states have mandatory rate-setting programs as low states, and the medium business states are equally distributed between the three categories of rate setting.

Because the first rate-setting programs began in the Northeast, it has been assumed that rate setting occurs only in eastern states. In fact, six of the ten states with mandatory programs are northeastern: Massachusetts, Maine, Connecticut, New York, New Jersey, and Maryland. But the four other states—West Virginia, Oregon, Washington, and Wisconsin—are scattered in the North Central, Mid-Atlantic, and Pacific/Mountain regions.

If there is no longer an indisputable geographic association with rate-setting policy solutions, there certainly has been a geographic association with the development of alternative delivery systems such as HMOs and PPOs, both generally considered to be competitive alternatives to rate setting as a way to control health care costs. HMOs and PPOs have been much more active in the Pacific, East North Central, and South Atlantic regions. In the FAH survey, questions were asked about the existence of PPOs in the various states. PPO development generally requires changes in state law or regulation to allow selective contracting with providers or weaker restrictions on freedom of choice of providers; thus, its passage would also require a strong challenge of existing provider interests. Once the business community and the insurance community in California supported the 1982 MediCal changes that allowed contracting with pre-

TABLE 9.3   *Existence of Rate-Setting Programs in 50 States by Levels of Business Participation, 1984 (in percentages)*

Rate Setting	High Business	Med. Business	Low Business	Total
None[a]	28	25	31	28
	(5)	(4)	(5)	(14)
Some[b]	56	50	56	54
	(10)	(8)	(9)	(27)
Yes[c]	16	31	13	18
	(3)	(4)	(2)	(9)
Total	100	100	100	100
	(18)	(16)	(16)	(50)

Sources: FAH Survey 1984; InterStudy Survey 1983.

Note: Measures of association are Chi square = 1.67
                        Effect parameter = + 0

[a]None = No mandatory rate-setting programs existed in the state.
[b]Some = Rate setting was being discussed, or there was voluntary rate review.
[c]Yes = Rate setting was mandatory for all payers.

ferred providers, the legislation passed quickly. In the FAH survey in 1984, thirty-nine states reported PPO activity underway or under consideration, and most of that activity was located in the medium or high participation states.

The geographic distribution shows none of the nine active PPO states located in the Northeast. On the surface this would seem to validate the conclusion that PPOs are more active outside the Northeast and more active in states without rate-setting programs. However, Connecticut, Florida, Maryland, New York, Washington, and Wisconsin, all states with rate-setting or review programs, showed some PPO development. Of the remainder of the rate-setting states, only Maine, New Jersey, and West Virginia showed no PPO development. The association of business activity and PPO activity may be clear, but the relationship between rate setting and PPO development needs more study.

What other health policy changes might be associated with business participation? In a previous study, I tested the association between business participation and various other health policy changes as described in the FAH survey, grouping the states according to the FAH, the Inter-Study, and the Chamber of Commerce of the U.S. categories of business participation. No matter how the states were grouped on their level of business participation, the positive direction of the associations remained the same, and the strength of the relationships remained essentially the same. That is, states with high business participation were much more likely than other states to have financial disclosure laws, state cost-containment commissions, and PPOs already in operation. States with high business participation were only somewhat more likely to have programs for the medically indigent, legislative changes toughening and strengthening health planning, and increases instead of cuts in their Medicaid programs in 1984, although increases or cuts in a single year tell very little of the story of the trajectory of those programs. As I have just demonstrated, there was no apparent relationship between the degrees of business participation in a state and the existence of state rate-setting programs.[22]

The obvious conclusion about the association of business participation and health policy change at the state level is that factors other than simply business participation contribute to policy change. It seems plausible that levels of urbanization, unionization, health care costs, state fiscal crisis, or even the type and number of corporations headquartered in the state could help account for these changes. Indeed, the previous study tested the impact of some of these "third" factors on the associations between business participation and financial disclosure. Although urbanization, level of hospital costs, and state fiscal crisis all showed strong associations with the existence of financial disclosure legislation in the states, no variable diminished the original association between business and financial disclosure. In states with high hospital costs, however, both business participation and costs appeared independently related to disclosure. Because hospital costs have been high in many of these states for years and business participation has been more recent, the level of costs may have been an important factor provoking business to seek the passage of financial disclosure laws. Certainly both case studies suggest that high health care costs and cost shifts to providers, provided the context in which business organized itself to promote policy change.[23]

Summary

The evidence from this fifty-state study supports and corroborates evidence from the two case studies as well as the study of federal policy making. Both Massachusetts and California were originally selected because of the visibility of their business participation and the high degree of policy innovation in 1982. Both states were demonstrably high in business participation, as well as in levels of urbanization, fiscal crisis, and hospital costs.

What explains the lack of business coalition activity and lack of policy change in the low participation states? As is evident from the map (Figure 9.1), the low participation states cluster most strongly in the Mountain and West North Central regions; they are also generally rural states with fewer large and active corporations. Rural states such as these, with little or no fiscal crisis and few organizations or centers of corporate power, tend to have less policy innovation and a greater centralization of power by a few, usually provider, interests. It is not difficult to imagine Idaho or Montana, with their hospital and physician associations dominating the state legislature, preventing the passage of financial disclosure laws. It is easy to picture a state in which there has been no political participation by business, however, changed by the emerging participation of business leaders in newly located centers of corporate power. In fact, the way single, dominant employers stimulated state-level policy change in Illinois and Iowa within the past few years demonstrates that possibility.

One more factor influencing change was not included in this study, but it presents an interesting object of further research. There has been substantial speculation about the impact and power of business or employer-only coalitions versus the more broad-based federations that include providers as voting members. Are employer-only coalitions more effective in promoting policy change? Do they tend to support any one type of policy change over another? Using the FAH and Chamber data, eighteen states emerged that had at least one employer-only coalition, and none of these states was in the low business participation category. Of these eighteen states, twelve were high business states, and four were medium participation states, indicating that the higher the level of business participation, the more likely employer-only groups will control the political process.

Although the FAH and Chamber data do not tie employer-only coalitions to patterns of policy change, a recent study of business coalitions by McLaughlin, Zellers, and Brown has attempted to make those links.[24] They noted that employer-only coalitions, as defined by voting membership, represented 45 percent of active coalitions in 1986. They concluded that employer-only coalitions were less fragile than broad-based ones; that they were more likely to focus on the promotion and creation of alternative delivery systems and less likely to engage only in educational activities; and that they viewed their role in the community as a leader as well as an educator.[25] The evidence in the surveys cited in this chapter supports these conclusions. Where business is active, no matter how one defines that activity, there is likely to be a matrix of policy aimed at changing the system and bringing health care costs down. And although economic and geographic factors contribute to levels and types of business participation, the political factor of business organization and participation and its impact on policy cannot be discounted.

10

Purchasing Alliances in Health

BUSINESS HAS BECOME an important political force in health care politics in the past twenty years. Even if health care costs moderate somewhat in the next decade, it is unlikely that business will withdraw from the policy process. The bottom line is, who cares? What difference has it made for business, politics, or policy?

Business ought to care because it is partially responsible for the continuing mess of escalating costs and irresponsible cost shifts. Policymakers ought to care because, lacking a historical understanding, they will continue to reinvent the same mistakes and make incremental and marginal policy changes decade after decade. Providers ought to care because they find themselves increasingly squeezed by business in its role as buyer, insurer, and trustee. Academics ought to care because the 1970s and 1980s have witnessed the entry of a new political actor into the health policy arena that deserves further scrutiny and explanation. Labor ought to care because the fat kid on the seesaw has grabbed hold of the policy agenda, and the initiative and balance need to be restored. Ordinary consumers ought to care because corporations are increasingly speaking in their names and their interests. And politicians and state officials ought to care because business can be an ally in producing structural change as well as a gatekeeper to the democratic process.

What do the cases described in this book and the questions raised mean? And what is likely to happen in the next decade?

Business and Health Care Politics

I believe that the evidence supports the conclusion that business was not very active in the 1960s when Medicare was passed, that it became more central to the policy debates of the 1970s and 1980s, and that few major health policies will be passed in the 1990s in which business interests are not represented and on which business does not have some impact. Business has organized a variety of both stable and fragile mechanisms for expressing its political interests. Some coalitions are unlikely to survive in their present form into the 1990s; state roundtables and lobbying groups such as the Washington Business Group on Health will persist.

Although economic crisis continues to be the most powerful motivator for business political participation, other political and cultural factors both promote and impede this participation. The degree of state regulatory activity, the general level of policy innovation, and prior levels of business activism in social policy can all affect current levels of business participation.[1] I have shown how the economic turbulence of the 1970s propelled business into awareness and action in health care; and I have also shown how moderating costs in the mid-1980s were associated with a slowdown in political activism. The late 1980s are filled with examples of reactivated health care task forces and new strategies for cost containment on the part of large corporations, as health insurance premiums rose an average of 20 percent between 1987 and 1988 and are expected to increase annually in the double digits well into the 1990s.[2]

The political participation of business in any policy arena is bound to be cyclical, waxing and waning with short-term results of short-term interventions. However, once organizations and alliances are formed, they have a life of their own. Present organizational effectiveness is always based on past challenges, and the challenges of the 1970s and 1980s to contain health care costs are not yet solved. Some type of political organization and mobilization, therefore, is bound to continue in the 1990s.

Furthermore, the continuing application of the econoimc paradigm in health care can only strengthen the political role of business, perhaps to its chagrin. The development of the American health care system is proceeding in the direction of greater efficiency, rationalization, and complexity. That trend is not likely to be reversed. Concurrently, the debate over health policy will continue to be developed within a language in which the market and economics define what will be considered "problems" (that is, the cost of health care more prominently than its distribution) as well as solutions (that is, all-payer systems or competing health plans, both choices that strengthen existing players and dominant ideologies).[3]

The market is viewed as a superior decision maker by policymakers because of the difficulty of making ethical or rationing choices in the political arena. "One of the greatest virtues of the market mechanism is its ability to relieve government of a myriad of complex and difficult decisions," such as who will get artificial hearts, who will live and who will die.[4] As Sheldon Wolin asserts, the political use of economics "is to mask power by presenting what are essentially political and moral questions in the form of economic choices. As the society moves from a condition of surplus to one of scarcity, economic policies are ways of distributing sacrifices."[5]

Within the dominance of this economically constructed reality, business has emerged as the appropriate political leader, with its impeccable ideological credentials of profit orientation and performance standards of efficiency. Business leaders, once reviled by the public, are now being asked to rescue the health care system from its irrationality and even its inequities. Republicans want to let the private sector do it all; Democrats at least want the private sector on the side of the state. The private sector itself, American business, has become the bride, and a somewhat reluctant one at that, in an arranged marriage to the state.

Aside from the very real problems of conducting the rescue, American business may not want to be the standard bearer or the arbiter of choices that are fundamentally political in nature. As Bob Burnett reminds us, health care cost containment is a dirty project.[6] It is filled with time-consuming meetings, rough policy fights, dangerous public exposure, and, even at best, considerable political risks for the participants. As business continues to participate politically, even sporadically, what impact will business have on the rest of the players on the seesaw? Will increased business power lead to increased power and participation of the other interests, or will the growth and complexity in the health care system itself be reflected in a similar complexity and fragmentation of the stakeholder interests?

Hospitals

In health care politics, hospitals are powerful interests, often major employers in their communities and states. Because a majority of the health care dollar continues to be spent in hospitals, hospitals are also the central focus of cost-containment efforts. As the health care system becomes corporatized, hospitals play an increasingly important role in managing and distributing resources. However, as hospital systems become more complex and gain legal and institutional power, they also inevitably fragment into component interests that better represent the regions, ownership, or specialty care provided. Just as one hospital association can no longer represent all hospitals, regionally or nationally, the power of any one association over the health policy agenda is lessened.

In the legislative arena, hospitals have reigned almost as supremely as physicians in most states. In Massachusetts, for example, the hospital lobby continues to be a significant force in legislative politics even though new associations have been formed to represent HMOs and teaching hospitals. In California, the old California Association of Hospitals has become the California Association of Hospitals and Health Systems and must now compete with regional hospital councils, an association of public hospitals, a for-profit hospital association,and powerful legislative advocates for the University of California teaching hospitals. Although most hospitals can still stop or modify legislation at the state level, they can no longer pass controversial legislation unilaterally.

Although business and hospital interests may occasionally coincide, business has several powerful points of leverage over hospitals: First, business representatives sit on hospital boards of trustees and have the potential to veto hospital behavior before it gets to the legislative level. Second, most nonhealth businesses continue to be more sensitive to their markets than hospitals. Business generally understands productivity and how to achieve it, but hospitals are only beginning to translate their service inputs and outputs into products and performance. And third, business has become, along with government, the principal client and purchaser of hospital services. Because most business purchasers have more market power than hospitals within regional markets, business as buyer continues to have the potential to control hospital as seller. Ultimately, hospitals and purchasers have strong congruent interests in rationalizing, economizing, and streamlining the hospital industry. They are both corporate rationalizers in Alford's terms, and their interests coincide much more powerfully than business purchasers and physician interests.

Insurers

The insurance industry is sluggish, conservative, and difficult to penetrate, even with the sharpest point of purchasing power. The largest insurers, both commercial and nonprofit, have resisted change in the health care system, preferring to rely on their legal and institutional power to keep their market share. The "unholy alliance" between insurers and hospitals that characterized the alliances of Blue Cross with hospitals and physicians around the country until the 1980s is beginning to break down.[7] Business purchasers have helped to break insurers away from hospitals. In Massachusetts, the commercial insurers and purchasers were firmly aligned in the Business Roundtable, and even Blue Cross of Massachusetts eventually broke away from the hospital association to "serve our customers" as they characterized Massachusetts business.

The close relationship between purchasers and insurers has not always been of benefit to purchasers, however. In Washington, D.C., in the early 1980s, the Chamber of Commerce was persuaded by the Reagan administration to separate purchaser from insurer interests on their health care task forces. And the presence of a Metropolitan Life executive as a representative of business on the Dunlop Group prompted some to call it "The Dunlop Group of Five" and others to acknowledge that the conflicts impede and dilute the effectiveness of the purchaser role. Despite these complexities, business has begun to recognize that insurers are potential allies and business has begun to exercise its muscle by forming alliances with insurance companies to control health care costs.

Physicians

Physicians, long the dominant force in health care politics, have lost both market and political power in the 1980s.[8] "If one attended a lot of medical meetings or read the letters columns of medical journals, one would have concluded that the physician's economic franchise was a smoking ruin, overrun and captured by the Huns of cost containment."[9] Forces such as the oversupply of physicians, the privatization and corporatization of health care, the increasing proportion of physicians in group rather than individual practice, information about physician practice and costs, and state policies regulating physician behavior are all factors contributing to the decline in political power.

In a Connecticut business coalition in 1987, information surfaced about differences in physician patterns of practice and charges. A physician member of the coalition, in an attempt to explain these variations, turned to a large employer and said, "You don't understand." "No," interrupted the employer. "*You* don't understand. The game is over."[10] And, indeed, by the end of the 1980s, the larger corporations had begun to understand just how medicine contributed to escalating health care costs. No longer were physician diagnoses or charges accepted without question. Although physician associations continued to be successful lobbying organizations at state and national levels, other forces in the health system were relentlessly reducing professional power.

Labor

The role of American labor in health care politics deserves a book of its own. I have not attempted to explain the unions' participation or lack thereof at either the state or national level, although I have tried to point out the policy consequences of leaving labor out of the debate. In some industrial states, such as Michigan or Illinois, where union activity is high, business has forged important alliances with labor. In other states, such as Iowa or Massachusetts, labor and management have found it difficult to establish common ground. As Bert Seidman of the AFL-CIO explained, "We have had to struggle to be acknowledged in the Reagan administration, and we do not expect that to change. However, we make sure we are heard on major national health issues in Congress, and we have made a major effort to educate labor people all over the country so we remain at the table." [11]

One national effort to promote the participation of labor has been the Dunlop Group of Six, in which three members of labor participate to one of every other interest. John Dunlop has explicitly augmented the participation of labor to strengthen the labor role in the national health policy discussion. Whether three members on Dunlop's group make up for the absence of labor in planning bodies across the country is doubtful. If labor were to increase its participation at the state and local level, its impact would be felt more readily at the national level. The power of management cannot be successfully exercised, however, without the participation of labor. As Seidman comments, "There will be no corporatism in the United States unless labor becomes stronger. Corporatism requires a strong labor representation."

Consumers

Consumers of health care (other than corporations) have been generally underrepresented on health care task forces or statewide commissions. Although representatives of the elderly and minorities were included on the Roberti Coalition in California, their influence depended on the leadership ability and skills of their members, not the organization of the constituencies they represented. The business members on the Roberti Coalition were backed by their respective regional coalitions and had the advantage of the concurrent lobbying support of the California Chamber of Commerce.

In Massachusetts, consumer members were not included on either the 1981 Joint Commission or the 1982 coalition. With the election of Michael Dukakis as governor in 1982, both consumer representatives and labor were assured participation in the commissions of the late 1980s. The effectiveness of the consumer member in the 1987 commission was a combination of the group of constituencies she had organized, as well as her personal skills and knowledge. Still, the business representative complained that she came to the table "without a checkbook." Business as buyer still had considerably more clout than individual consumer as buyer when it came to controlling behind-the-scenes politics. The consumer groups remained effective by allying themselves with business and the state, and to a lesser degree by manipulating the media through demonstrations and rallies. In the 1990s, organized citizen groups may find themselves turning to the statewide political initiative as a tool to increase their political power.

The State

Business has reinforced and reproduced its power through alliance with the state. In both the state case studies the state brought business into the policy process. State officials organized business participation in the joint commission in Massachusetts and the Roberti Coalition in California, and state officials in Washington organized business into the national policy task forces in order to augment state power. The combined purchasing power of the state and business caused considerable structural change in health policy in both Massachusetts and California.

If the state shifts its basis of legitimacy from its role as guardian of the public interest to negotiator of technical expertise with private elites, however, state power could ultimately be diminished. In the late 1980s, the state of Massachusetts, in alliance with business, had an opportunity to exercise considerable power. It did so, passing the first comprehensive health insurance legislation in the country. However, the state also had the opportunity to create a new state agency that would have combined all purchasing power of the state into one entity, a concentration of power that was too threatening a demonstration of state power to survive.

Business and the Policy Process

There have been genuine changes in the policy process in the 1980s, not just in health. At both the state and national level, varying degrees of fiscal crisis have provided the state with the opportunity to insert a thin wedge of structural change. Several factors have contributed to substantial policy changes in the policy process and its outcomes: using the budget reconciliation process as a Trojan horse filled with a variety of reform proposals; combining symbolic public commissions and the privatization of agenda formation; removing decisions from the political arena to the economic realm with the powerful sledge hammer of market ideology; and delegating decisions from the federal to the state level, thereby fragmenting political opposition into fifty centers.

The role of business in the health policy process has strengthened and been strengthened by each of these trends. Elite interests are not always served by the Trojan horse approach (e.g., passage of the 1986 COBRA extension of benefits for workers was opposed by business, and cost shifts to business from Medicare and Medicaid have continued), but on balance consolidating state power usually provokes a reaction from business and can ultimately increase the exercise of private power. In combination with private negotiations, public participation by business elites can reinforce and reproduce business power.

Decision making by the market is not always favored by business because the control of health care costs depends on being able to squeeze all parts of the balloon. Still, business knows how to manipulate markets and when decision making becomes stalemated in the political arena, as it has in the past, fragmenting those decisions into dozens of buying and selling decisions can benefit buyers who have some consolidated purchasing power. In Arizona, when business failed to manipulate the political process and lost its legislative initiative campaign, it was forced to fall back on market solutions of HMOs and PPOs, which, as business leaders pointed out, might solve cost problems for individual companies but did not contain overall costs in the system.

Decentralizing political power to the state level removes policy issues from central national attention or debate. National Health Insurance did not occur in the 1980s; Massachusetts comprehensive health insurance did. While a national commission debated reform of physician fees, Massachusetts passed a law forbidding physicians to bill patients for more than Medicare would reimburse. Reform and change have been most dramatic at the state level in the 1980s, where business elites have considerable power and access. For multistate and multinational employers, however, a national policy solution may be preferable to policy reform in fifty different locations. The 1990s may bring the debate back to the national level.

Points of Access in the Policy Process

There is little debate over the ability of business elites to gain access to the policy process, but at what points of the process will business be most effective? Clarence Stone has noted in his study of urban policy in Atlanta that business demands had the most impact at exactly those points where electoral demands were weakest: that is, business had power where issues originated and where they were implemented. Business demands were least effective at the point of decision by elected officials.[12] I have shown examples of business participation in the formation of the policy agenda through the Washington, D.C., policy advisory groups, the WBGH's input into data disclosure legislation and physician antitrust legislation, the Massachusetts Business Roundtable's private legislative process, and the collaboration of the business membership on the Roberti Coalition and California Chamber of Commerce in feeding policy ideas to state decision makers. Although business has extraordinary access to the policy process when it chooses to make demands, business leadership tends to deny its impact. As the *Harvard Business Review* reminds its readers, "The business community has been anything but a major player in the agenda-setting arena. . . . Business and industry frequently are 'reactive.'"[13]

Staying involved in the implementation phase of policy requires a highly unified business group. Business power was exercised to maintain the gains in implementing MediCal reform in California in 1983 and 1984, despite efforts by the providers to overturn the contracting aspects of the legislation. California business leaders continued to keep their coalitions together throughout the 1980s, hiring lobbyists, monitoring legislation, and even introducing their own bills as challenges emerged to business gains.

The point at which decisions are made in the legislative process is the weakest point of entry for business demands. Although business leaders have learned to play the legislative game in some states, they have failed rather visibly in others. In Arizona, the leaders of the business coalitions were engineers. "The [political] initiatives were drafted with the same precision that went into developing the jet airplane, and with the same kind of logic. . . . This turned out to be the coalition's fundamental error: its leaders neglected political considerations when designing the initiatives. For all the plan's exactness, it could not be compromised, and . . . could not fly in turbulent political air."[14] The appearance at hearings, letter writing campaigns, skill in negotiating out political settlements, and courting of politicians are usually neither part of a CEO's repertoire of skills nor high on a corporate leader's agenda.

Business Alliances for Health

One *Harvard Business Review* suggestion to business leaders who want more legislative impact is to establish networks and alliances. Business learned that lesson in health policy in the 1980s. Of all potential alliances, the alliance of public and private purchasers had the most promise but the least stability. The fragile or potential corporatism that characterized the private planning process in Massachusetts fits within a limited definition of corporatism: a strong state presence, a two-way policy process, organized constituencies, and public ratification of private decisions. By the late 1980s, the state role remained strong and had even been strengthened, but the demands of broader consumer groups fragmented elite control, constituencies melted, and the legislature more aggressively took back its responsibility for policy decisions. This limited corporatist planning has worked best in a state such as Massachusetts, where the geographic area and the number of participants is small and where there is a history and acceptance of a strong state regulatory role. Even though this type of concentrated planning may not have occurred in quite the same way in other states, the activist role of the state in California and Massachusetts demands that an interpretation of the policy process include the state as a critical actor and an interest in and of itself.

The alliance of business with other interests is more common and more permanent, although to the degree that business becomes just another interest among a medley of providers, it can lose the impact of its concentrated purchasing power. The promotion of multiparty business and health coalitions by the Robert Wood Johnson Foundation and the Dunlop Group may have diluted the effective use of business power because of the inherent instability of such coalitions.[15]

In order to promote and pass legislation, business often develops alliances with insurers or providers. Alliances with nonprofit sector providers have the potential to lend legitimacy to business power and decrease distrust and fear of the abuse of private power. By the end of the 1980s, however, the legitimacy of the nonprofit sector was questioned and legally challenged, primarily because of decreasing differences in organizational behavior between for-profit and nonprofit providers.[16] It no longer became an automatic advantage for business to ally itself with the nonprofit sector, per se, unless the alliance took advantage of the market power of that sector. In the East and Midwest, where penetration by for-profit insurers and providers was less than in the West and Southwest, business was likely to make alliances with whatever groups dominated the market, regardless of their tax status.

An alliance of business and labor is both the most natural and the most difficult of all alliances. At the national level, where labor's political clout is strongest, alliances such as the Labor-Management Group, an informal group that met actively in the 1970s, served to promote shared agendas in a powerful way. The Dunlop Group, structured as it was to favor labor interests, was also a place where business and labor could form alliances, and, although the Dunlop Group has had no demonstrated or specifiable impact on health policy thus far, the commonality of interest between the business and labor members has been noted by the other members. As Bert Seidman of the AFL-CIO has commented, "In reading over the Labor-Management Group policy statements on health care in 1977 and 1987, I am surprised to see how much we agreed then, as well as now. Except for a few issues, we're together."[17]

The Privatization of the Policy Process

Although business has found it convenient to operate in a policy environment that is private, using business style negotiations and bargaining among the interests, this mode of policymaking is by no means the normal public context. A Business Roundtable report concludes, "Little in [executive] education or business experience prepares them for participation in the untidy and often bruising public policy process."[18] In instances such as the Massachusetts negotiations, where business was able to conduct the policy discussions in private with preselected and invited participants, business could control the agenda and the policy process. In California, business was by no means dominant, and the bruising process of the Roberti Coalition finally drove business leaders to meet in private to formulate their strategy.

If business controls the policy process best when it becomes involved in agenda setting and can make alliances with the state and other interests, business also exercises control when it can define its interests as equivalent to consumer interests. In California, business was identified as representing all buyers when it put the squeeze on physicians, but not even all organized buyers were involved, much less the unorganized consumer constituencies not represented by corporations. What is the consumer interest in health care? Because business can write a large check, it becomes, by default, the consumer buyer, but there are many pitfalls to reinforcing the purchasers in this role.

One problem with large corporations acting as agents for their employees (or even large unions) is whether the "paternalistic corporation" will demand and get effective information and whether employees can interpret that information to promote health or only cost containment. Robert Evans, the Canadian economist notes, "There is no basis for any a priori assumption that in a highly 'information-impacted' environment the result will be a more effective, much less a more cost-effective health care system."[19] The experience of cost containment in the 1980s has been an experience of massive shifts in cost responsibility from public to private sectors and from management to employees. Medicare saves money by paying hospitals less and imposing higher co-payments on the elderly; companies save money by increasing deductibles and copayments for their employees; employees save money by not seeking care. None of these shifts promotes better health.

To the extent that business has successfully promoted the privatization and occasionally dominated the policy process in health, these consequences have profoundly antidemocratic implications. This type of powerful alliance has led many scholars to conclude that the fusion of public and private power can be dangerous to democracy and the representative political process.[20] The concentration of too much power in either state or private entities is generally feared and avoided. The European experience with the fusion of public and private power through corporatist planning mechanisms has been predicted for the United

States, but so far only the most fragile moments of fusion have been created by moments of crisis. Under conditions of state fiscal crisis, the policy process was captured by private interests in Massachusetts and directed largely by public interests in California. Observers are left without any clear trend but with the sense that in situations of crisis, both the state and business have the power, when united, to break provider monopoly over policy and create structural change. Whether these alliances will endure remains to be seen in the next decade.

Substantive Policy Change

A final word on the substance of policy change. This book is filled with examples of the pragmatism of business in its selection of policy solutions. The case studies show California and Massachusetts business leaders supporting polar opposite policy solutions to similar policy problems. The fifty-state study shows strong business participation associated with the release and availability of data and information about health care costs but no pattern over the support of regulating the health care system. Does that mean that business has had no impact on the substance of health policy? Business leaders in Iowa were the primary force for financial disclosure of hospital costs and charges; in Massachusetts they were the force for regulating hospital costs. Although the patterns are not consistent, the association of business participation with substantive change is clear. Within the context of the dominant market ideology of the 1980s, business support for alternative delivery systems, more and better data, utilization control, and occasionally rate regulation, has often been the force that tipped the balance away from the status quo.

The Power of Business as a Purchaser of Health Care

I come finally to the most difficult question of all. Of what does the power of business consist? Under what conditions can business most successfully exercise its power, and what might happen if business did exercise that power?

What is business power? As demonstrated in Massachusetts, it is the power to move a plant out of the state, to hire and fire and produce wealth, to form political organizations to express interests, to have extraordinary access to influential decision makers and the ideas that produce change. It is not the power to produce change from acting alone in the political arena. It is the power to forge alliances and consensus among many interests and act as a catalyst to force policy change on a stagnant or stubborn political system.

Under what conditions are these various levels of power successfully exercised? Business will obviously exercise its power most successfully when the many factions of business are unified. Because perfect unity is unlikely, one should take another look at the situations in which business interests were unified or fragmented and try to understand how that fragmentation affected the successful exercise of business power.

Many types of conflict undermine unity between segments of business: conflicts between business, big and small; between business as buyer and provider of health care; between business as purchaser and as hospital trustee; and between purchasers and insurers. There are also significant differences between large and small organizations in the orientation of the firm to the outside world and the internal resources available to solve problems. In Massachusetts, the Business Roundtable represented big business in Massachusetts. It fell to the Massachusetts Chamber of Commerce to represent small business, and I have shown that the Chamber was not central in the policy discussions. When Governor Dukakis passed his "health care for all" legislation in mid-1988, it was structured to benefit big business. Small businesses bore the brunt of the cost of the new taxes, but their protests did nothing to stop the legislation.

By 1988, the Massachusetts Business Roundtable represented mainly stable manufacturing companies, commercial insurers, and utility companies. The newer high technology companies had broken away to form their own autonomous business group. It is difficult to estimate how this fragmentation affected business in the legislative arena. The other interests had fragmented, too, and there were several new participants in the policy process: labor and consumers. As a consequence of internal fragmentation within the business groups and the proliferation of new interests, the domination of business at the legislative level in Massachusetts had been reduced from its high point in 1982.

Conflicts between business as buyer and provider have been noted in the way coalitions structured themselves as employer-only or multiparty, and as health-related or non-health-related business. Although provider organizations are also buyers of health insurance for their employees, I have not included them as examples of purchasing power in health because of the obvious conflicts in goals and approaches to cost containment that might surface. The Arizona situation provides one major example where a health-related business was unable to forcefully exercise its purchasing power because of these conflicts.

When business first awoke to rising health care costs in Arizona, the four major employers in the state were involved: Sperry, Motorola, Garrett, and Honeywell corporations. When the conflict between hospitals and business escalated to the political initiative stage, the hospital association took out an ad in *The Wall Street Journal* warning other businesses about "all-out corporate warfare" and what they called "legislative terrorism."[21] Because Honeywell supplied computer equipment to hospitals all over the country, Honeywell began receiving canceled contracts from hospitals in Arizona as well as elsewhere. The corporate headquarters of Honeywell requested that the Arizona plant CEO withdraw from the coalition, and he did. The relationship of business type to political participation has been little studied, but it seems clear that to the extent that a company has few or no ties with the health care industry, it will be able to bargain more effectively with health care providers.

The conflict that a purchaser representative discovers when he tries to wear the hat of hospital trustee is far from resolved. Once characterized as "checking their brains at the door," business representatives who sit on hospital boards often face tricky and uncomfortable divided loyalties. In the heat of the Massachusetts negotiations in 1982, the Roundtable members used their hospital board affiliations to control hospital behavior in the coalition, but not all the members understood their leverage. In 1987, the executive director of the Roundtable recalled a hospital board meeting where he was asked to contribute to a hospital lobbying fund to oppose a bill that the Roundtable was supporting. "Why would I shoot myself in my own backside?" he asked exasperatedly. Yet, a number of the Roundtable business members did contribute to the fund, apparently not recognizing the rather clear contradictions.

Within business another type of conflict surfaced at the national and state level over the relationship of purchasers and insurers. At the national Business Roundtable, Metropolitan Life Chairman John Creedon has been the head of the Health Care Task Force for the past several years. He also sits as a representative of business to the Dunlop Group of Six. The conflicts between his role as insurer and purchaser are noted by his staff and other members, and it is generally accepted that a business representative with no ties to the industry could represent business more forcefully. The very care with which Creedon approaches issues, however, probably dilutes the successful exercise of business power. If he were to have to leave the room during a discussion, as he has promised to do if a conflict arises, no business point of view would be represented.

The relationship of commercial insurers and purchasers on the MBRT in Massachusetts represented a complex merger of interests. Commercial insurers wanted the Roundtable to participate in health policy because the insurers wanted a larger share of the Massachusetts health insurance market. The fact that insurers were a fifth of the Roundtable board of directors influenced the Roundtable's decision to pursue a regulatory strategy and made it more difficult for Nelson Gifford to represent himself persuasively as a neutral, honest broker for business interests in general.

These examples are reminders that business can most successfully exercise its purchasing power when business segments are unified and when the role of business as purchaser is not in direct conflict with the role of business as provider, supplier, or trustee.

Another condition that enhances the exercise of business power is the size of the firm participating in the policy debate, its market power, and the role of its CEO. I have already described the clout that three of the four largest manufacturers in Arizona were able to wield. In Iowa, John Deere and Company, one of the largest employers in the state, was able to make alliances with several other large employers, including the *Des Moines Tribune*, and produce an unquestionable business presence in state health care politics in the early 1980s.

To note the presence and effectiveness of a few CEOs or large companies is not to deny that these may be exceptional cases. Most business coalitions and employer representatives are not CEOs; most are middle-management personnel or vice presidents of benefits. And even when a CEO participates in health policy discussions, that participation has its own half-life. As Lawrence Brown and Catherine McLaughlin noted in a study of twenty-one business coalitions, less than half were CEO-dominated, and only one was a "cohesive, meta coalition," capable of producing substantial community health system change. They did not find evidence of a corporate revolution in health care in their work, commenting instead, "There are good reasons . . . why corporate 'giants' and peers of lesser stature slept so long, now awaken slowly and fitfully, and sometimes prefer to switch off the alarm, roll over, and slumber anew." They also acknowledged, however, that when power is concentrated in the hands of a few payers, there is potential for generating significant reforms.[22]

Business and the Future of Purchasing Power

I have been considering the conditions under which purchasing power can be successfully exercised. It is acknowledged by all the major actors in health care politics that business does not always exercise its various levels of power to change the health care system. From the point of view of providers and other actors in health care politics, the worst thing that could happen if business truly exercised its purchasing power or, in the terms of one observer, "really played hard ball,"[23] ranges from extreme rationing of care to a total breakdown in the economic system.

Jim Sammons of the AMA notes, "The most negative potential of business participation in health care is if business started telling us how to treat our patients, or if American business became so marginal that it couldn't afford to pay for health care for its employees. Then we would all be in trouble, not just the purchsers."[24] Alexander Williams, vice president of the AHA, comments, "Playing hard ball requires top level, intense focus on a problem, and even at these prices is it worth that attention from a CEO? Let's suppose business plays hard ball, and by that I mean institutes draconian reductions in the amount of money being spent on health care. And let's suppose that significant changes are made. What are the unintended consequences? We've always had this expectation that we can do whatever we want with our health and the health care system will be there waiting to fix us up. If we rationed care too much, business could get out too far in front of the rest of society."[25] It seems unlikely that American business will ever push its power that far.

Trends in Health Care Politics for the 1990s

Given all these constraints, I can predict several trends about business participation in health care politics in the 1990s:

1. Health care costs are already increasing again with a vengeance. Although there was a dip in employer contributions to worker health insurance in 1984 and although there were some government savings in Medicare from the implementation of prospective payment in 1983, the overall evidence indicates that "both prices and real health expenditures have exploded since 1980." Recent national surveys have found that employers' health care costs are rising between 8 and 15 percent a year in the late 1980s, with some self-insured plans increasing as much as 25 to 40 percent in one year.[26]

2. Business will begin to participate again but in different forms, depending on the state and the previous experience of business in that state. "Employers were getting used to health costs going up only 5 percent to 7 percent a year," noted one expert. "If premiums start increasing by 10 percent or 12 percent a year, the club will come out of the closet.[27] "Employers are saying, 'That's it, we're not paying any more' because they can't pay any more."[28]

3. Business will go through stages of participation. As Edward Hennessy, Jr., of Allied-Signal, Inc., noted in *The Wall Street Journal* in 1988, "Unfortunately, most companies purchasing health care still aren't cost-conscious buyers—and those that are haven't yet taken steps to use their bargaining power effectively."[29] Not all businesses will go through all stages, however. Depending on the type, size, and location of the business, various stages will be more appropriate than others:

STAGE ONE: Education and awareness. All sizes and types of business begin at this stage, although the smaller the business, the more likely it is to remain here because of its lack of expertise and market leverage. This is the stage of endless lunches and meetings, of decisions about whether to remain an employer-only coalition or allow providers in to help interpret data, of collecting and refining data. If a business has been involved in an information-gathering coalition in the 1980s, it is not likely to remain at this stage in the 1990s.

STAGE TWO: The creation of new organizations or the reactivation of old ones. If a group of employers has not started a business and health coalition in their community, they will be likely to start one in the 1990s. If they had a coalition and disbanded it, they will be likely to move directly to the third and fourth stage. Mid-sized companies will be more likely to form new coalitions than large companies, which will be more likely to revitalize existing organizations.

STAGE THREE: Internal company strategies to reduce costs. Although utilization management, preadmission certification, increased deductibles and copayments, alternative delivery systems, and changes in benefit design have been common cost-containment solutions among large companies, smaller and mid-sized companies are just beginning to explore these options in the late 1980s. In Kansas City, a study of cost-containment programs of business and labor groups conducted by Mercer Meidinger Hansen and the Mid-America Coalition in 1988 discovered that, although utilization review programs were the most popular cost-containment method for most companies, 60 percent of the companies were unsure of the effectiveness of these programs.[30] The 1990s will see the use of all of these internal strategies as well as external pressure on the provider delivery system. Dr. Sammons predicts, "Business's next generation strategy will be more cost shifting to employees and more reductions in benefits. They will never become inactive now. It would be a big mistake to go back to the passive stance of the 1950s and 1960s."

STAGE FOUR: External purchasing alliances. "The leading industries will put the risk on the providers and move toward vertical integrated systems and capitation. This will be done through purchasing alliances."[31] Hennessy of Allied-Signal also notes, "Most company cost-containment programs have been futile because they've focused only on influencing consumers of health care. . . . The only way to achieve meaningful cost control [is] to give providers themselves a reason to work for this goal."[32] In Denver, Colorado, a group of employers have banded together in a "cooperative" with an employee base of 30,000 and a dependent base of 100,000. In San Diego, a cooperative of employers has 350,000 employees and dependents and has bargained for 35 to 40 percent discounts on hospital and physician bills from local providers.[33]

Purchasers will make alliances and use their market leverage on hospitals, particularly where there is a monopsony situation, with many sellers and only a few buyers. However, even if purchaser alliances successfully reduce rates for their own members, this will not mean cost savings in the health care system as a whole.

STAGE FIVE: Comprehensive solutions such as national or state-level health insurance, rate regulation or review, or powerful business-state alliances. This stage is neither inevitable, nor will it occur unless there is significant economic or political crisis in the system. Comprehensive solutions require extraordinary political effort and/or extraordinary economic strain. Some observers have noted that the central dynamic of the so-called "health care revolution of the 1980s" has been the shifting of economic power away from providers toward payers and an accompanying shift of economic risk from public and private payers to patients, physicians, and hospitals.[34]

Only if small business recognizes the cost shift from big business and refuses to accept it, if employees recognize the cost shift from employers and refuse to pay it, or if private payers recognize the cost shift from public programs and refuse to sanction it, will a comprehensive solution be workable or even likely. The "violent tremor in the health economy"[35] predicted for the 1990s may end up like the tremors predicted along the San Andreas fault in California. A series of smaller quakes may shake out the tension in the system but require no strong response, or one or two larger quakes may force action. Whatever the outcome, the purchasers of care, both business and the state, will be the major countervailing political force in the policy process.

APPENDIX A

Three Measures of Business Participation and Final Grouping of Fifty States

STATE	FAH	CHAMBER	INTERSTUDY	FINAL
Alabama	2	2	1	2
Alaska	1	2	1	1
Arizona	3	3	3	3
Arkansas	1	1	1	1
California	2	3	3	3
Colorado	2	2	1	2
Connecticut	3	2	3	3
Delaware	2	2	2	2
Florida	3	3	3	3
Georgia	2	2	2	2
Hawaii	2	2	2	2
Idaho	1	1	1	1
Illinois	2	3	3	3
Indiana	3	3	2	3
Iowa	3	3	2	3
Kansas	3	2	3	3
Kentucky[a]	1	3	2	2
Louisiana	1	1	1	1
Maine	1	1	2	1
Maryland	2	2	2	2
Massachusetts	3	3	3	3
Michigan	3	2	3	3
Minnesota[a]	1	2	3	2
Mississippi	1	1	1	1
Missouri	3	2	3	3
Montana	1	1	1	1
Nebraska	1	1	1	1
Nevada	2	1	1	1
New Hampshire	2	1	1	1
New Jersey	1	2	2	2
New Mexico	1	1	1	1
New York	3	3	3	3
North Carolina	3	3	2	3
North Dakota	1	1	1	1
Ohio	3	3	3	3
Oklahoma	3	3	1	3
Oregon	2	1	2	2
Pennsylvania	3	3	3	3
Rhode Island	2	1	1	1

APPENDIX A (*continued*)

STATE	FAH	CHAMBER	INTERSTUDY	FINAL
South Carolina	3	3	1	3
South Dakota	1	1	1	1
Tennessee	3	3	1	3
Texas[a]	2	3	1	2
Utah	3	2	2	2
Vermont	2	2	2	2
Virginia	2	2	—	2
Washington	2	2	2	2
West Virginia	1	1	2	1
Wisconsin	3	2	2	2
Wyoming	1	2	1	1

Measures of Participation: 1 = low business
                                                participation
                              2 = medium business
                                                participation
                              3 = high business
                                                participation

Sources: FAH Survey 1984; U.S. Chamber of Commerce Survey 1984; InterStudy Survey 1983.

[a]States on which there was no agreement as to category; final assigned measurement was 2, medium business participation.

APPENDIX B

List of States by Levels of Business Participation and Existence of Financial Disclosure Laws, 1984

FINANCIAL DISCLOSURE LEGISLATION	HIGH BUSINESS	MED. BUSINESS	LOW BUSINESS
NONE	Oklahoma California	Delaware Texas	Alaska Mississippi Montana New Mexico North Dakota Rhode Island South Dakota West Virginia
SOME	Michigan North Carolina Ohio Pennsylvania South Carolina Tennessee	Alabama Colorado Kentucky Minnesota Oregon Utah Wisconsin	Arkansas Idaho Louisiana Nebraska New Hampshire Wyoming
YES	Arizona Connecticut Florida Illinois Indiana Iowa Kansas Massachusetts Missouri New York	Georgia Hawaii Maryland New Jersey Vermont Virginia Washington	Maine Nevada

Sources: FAH Survey 1984; InterStudy Survey 1983.

APPENDIX C

List of States with Rate-Setting Programs by Levels of Business Participation, 1984

RATE SETTING LEGISLATION	HIGH BUSINESS	MED. BUSINESS	LOW BUSINESS
NONE	California Iowa Missouri Oklahoma South Carolina	Colorado Delaware Texas Alabama	Louisiana Mississippi Nebraska New Mexico North Dakota
SOME	Arizona Illinois Michigan Florida Indiana North Carolina Ohio Pennsylvania Tennessee	Oregon Georgia Hawaii Minnesota Kentucky Virginia Utah Vermont	Alaska Arkansas Idaho Montana Nevada New Hampshire South Dakota Wyoming Rhode Island
YES	Massachusetts Connecticut New York	Maryland Washington Wisconsin New Jersey	Maine West Virginia

Sources: FAH Survey 1984; InterStudy Survey 1983.

Notes

Chapter One: Business and Health Care Politics

1. Robert R. Alford, *Health Care Politics, Ideological and Interest Group Barriers to Reform* (Chicago: University of Chicago Press, 1975). Alford does not argue the impossibility of change but simply that extraordinary structures and events are necessary to break the usual stalemated health care politics.
2. See the discussion in Chapters 5 and 9 that explain the way the prospective payment policy was formulated, implemented, and supported or opposed by the various interest groups in the 1980s. For a thorough discussion of the changes in public- and private-sector policy in the past ten years, see the entire volume of *Journal of Health Politics, Policy and Law* 13:2 (Summer 1988), entitled "Competition in the Health Care Sector: Ten Years Later," Warren Greenberg, guest editor; Lawrence Brown, "Introduction to a Decade of Transition," *Journal of Health Politics, Policy and Law* 11:4 (1986):580; and Clark Havighurst, "The Changing Locus of Decision Making in the Health Care Sector," ibid., 712.
3. This is Paul Starr's term in *The Social Transformation of American Medicine* (New York: Basic Books, 1982), 378.
4. See Chapter 6 for a description of physician perceptions about business power and the reason physicians felt like "crabs in a bucket."
5. This term is used by Thomas Donahue, vice president for membership of the U.S. Chamber of Commerce, in Richard I. Kirkland, Jr., "Fat Days for the Chamber of Commerce," *Fortune* (21 September 1981):154.
6. These comments of Secretary Finch are quoted in Edmund Faltermayer, "Better Care at Less Cost Without Miracles," *Fortune* (January 1970):127.
7. Those businesses that provide medical care services or insure for medical care are not the focus of this study, even though all providers and insurers are also purchasers for their own employees and many corporations have subsidiaries that provide or insure for medical care. Businesses acting politically at the state or national level in the early 1980s mainly represented business as a purchaser or

buyer and attempted to distinguish themselves, either explicitly or implicitly, from provider businesses by labeling them vendors of medical care. The distinctions between purchasers and vendors are not neatly defined, however, and there are conflicts and divisions among business leaders over these distinctions.

8.   Jack Shelton, Ford Motor Company, as quoted in testimony before the Joint Economic Committee of the U.S. Congress, Washington, D.C., 12 April 1984.

9.   Linda Demkovich, "Business as a Health Care Consumer is Paying Heed to the Bottom Line," *National Journal* (24 May 1980):851–854; and "A Foster Higgins Health Care Benefits Survey, 1987," *Medical Benefits* (29 February 1988): 1–2.

10.   Joseph Califano, *America's Health Care Revolution* (New York: Random House, 1986), 31.

11.   The number of business and health coalitions in the United States is not easy to determine. In 1986, the Chamber of Commerce of the U.S. turned over its coalition data responsibility to the AHA, which began surveying coalitions on behalf of the Dunlop Group of Six (Business Roundtable, AFL-CIO, AHA, AMA, Blue Cross and Blue Shield Association, HIAA). The data base established by the AHA received surveys from 129 operational coalitions in forty-four states at the end of 1987. A resurvey in 1986 of all 215 active coalitions listed by the AHA in their 1985–1986 data base by an evaluation team (Catherine McLaughlin and Lawrence Brown) from the University of Michigan resulted in the location of thirty-five defunct coalitions, leaving a total of 178 active and operational coalitions in forty-six states at the end of 1986. The resurvey also confirmed from the coalition leaders themselves that 45 percent were "business only," while the AHA data base listed only 9.3 percent. These discrepancies will be discussed in later chapters. Because the evaluation team, sponsored by the Robert Wood Johnson Foundation, called every coalition, whereas the AHA relied on the return of a mail survey, I am using the evaluation's team numbers as the more up-to-date and accurate.

12.   Robert A. Burnett, the CEO of Meredith Corporation, as quoted in John K. Iglehart, "Big Business and Health Care in the Heartland: An Interview with Robert Burnett," *Health Affairs* 3:1 (Spring 1984):40–49.

13.   Committee for Economic Development, "Building a National Health Care System" (New York: Committee for Economic Development, April 1973), 90.

14.   Joseph Califano, "Can We Afford One Trillion for Health Care?" (Remarks to the Economic Club of Detroit, Michigan, 25 April 1983).

15.   John Crosier, as quoted in Jane Stein, "Bay State Employers' Role in the Health Care Arena," *Business and Health* 3:4 (March 1986):49.

16.   Ibid.

17.   Linda Demkovich, "Businesses Drive to Curb Medical Costs Without Much Help from Government," *National Journal* (11 August 1984):1508; and Executive Summary, "Joint State and Corporate Strategies to Reduce Health Cost Escalation," Proceedings of a conference in Boulder, Colorado, 16 January 1984 (Washington, D.C.: Washington Business Group on Health, February 1984), 2.

18.   A quote from Bob Burnett in John Iglehart's, "Big Business and Health Care in the Heartland," 43; also see Marilyn Musser and Sal Bognanni, "Coalition Spirit in Iowa Cements Health System Reform," *Business and Health* 1:5 (April 1984):37.

19. Interview with Bob Lee, vice president of Plantronics, Inc., in Santa Cruz, Calif., 25 May 1988.

20. Edward L. Hennessy, Jr., "A Completely New Way to Purchase Medical Benefits," *The Wall Street Journal* (18 July 1988); telephone interview with Joe Duva, corporate director of employee benefits for Allied-Signal, 1 August 1988.

21. Interview with Willis Goldbeck, president of the Washington Business Group on Health, in Washington, D.C., June 1984.

22. E. E. Schattschneider, *The Semisovereign People: A Realist's View of Democracy in America* (Hinsdale, Ill.: Dryden Press, 1960), 30.

23. These interventions are modeled after those described in the work of Michael Useem, *The Inner Circle: Large Corporations and the Rise of Business Political Activity in the U.S. and U.K.* (New York: Oxford University Press, 1984), 76.

24. The fragmentation argument is put forth by academics such as John T. Dunlop, *Business and Public Policy* (Cambridge: Harvard University Press, 1980), 103; and Leonard Silk and David Vogel, *Ethics and Profits: The Crisis of Confidence in American Business* (New York: Simon and Schuster, 1976), 181. Proponents of a view that business power is more concentrated include Ralph Miliband, *The State in Capitalist Society* (New York: Basic Books, 1969); William G. Domhoff, *Who Rules America?* (Englewood Cliffs, N.J.: Prentice-Hall, 1967); Domhoff, *The Higher Circles: The Governing Class in America* (New York: Random House, 1970); Domhoff, *The Powers That Be: Process of Ruling Class Domination in America* (New York: Random House, 1979); Domhoff, *Who Rules America Now? A View for the '80s* (New York: Simon and Schuster, 1983); and J. Allen Whitt, "Can Capitalists Organize Themselves?" in *Power Structure Research*, ed. W. G. Domhoff (Beverly Hills, Calif.: Sage, 1980), 97–114.

25. Useem, *The Inner Circle*, 6.

26. Regina Herzlinger, "How Companies Tackle Health Care Costs, Part II," *Harvard Business Review* 63:5 (September–October 1985):120.

27. See Harvey Sapolsky, Drew Altman, Richard Green, and Judith Moore, "Corporate Attitudes Toward Health Care Costs," *Milbank Memorial Fund Quarterly/Health and Society* 59:4 (1981):560–585, for the best-known refutation of corporate interest and involvement in health care activities.

28. Raymond Bauer, Ithiel de Sola Pool, and Lewis Dexter, *American Business and Public Policy: The Politics of Foreign Trade*. 2d ed. (New York: Atherton Press, 1972), 487.

29. Graham K. Wilson, *Business and Politics: A Comparative Introduction* (London: Macmillan, 1985), 30.

Chapter Two: Power, Policy, and Politics

1. Robert A. Dahl, "The Concept of Power," in *Political Power: A Reader in Theory and Research*, ed. Roderick Bell, David M. Edwards, R. Harrison Wagner (New York: Free Press, 1969); and Nelson W. Polsby, *Community Power and Political Theory* (New Haven, Conn.: Yale University Press, 1963). These authors are also cited by John Gaventa, *Power and Powerlessness: Quiescence and*

Rebellion in an Appalachian Valley (Chicago: University of Illinois Press, 1980), 5.

2. Charles E. Lindblom, *Politics and Markets: The World's Political-Economic Systems* (New York: Basic Books, 1977), 356.

3. For a full explanation of these units of analysis and levels of power, see Robert Alford and Roger Friedland, *Powers of Theory, Capitalism, the State, and Democracy* (New York: Cambridge University Press, 1985).

4. Peter Bachrach and Morton Baratz, "The Two Faces of Power," *American Political Science Review* 56 (1962):947–952; Schattschneider, *Semisovereign People.*

5. Matthew A. Crenson, *The Un-Politics of Air Pollution: A Study of Non-Decision Making in the Cities* (Baltimore: Johns Hopkins University Press, 1971).

6. Steven Lukes, *Power: A Radical View* (London: Macmillan, 1974).

7. Gaventa, *Power and Powerlessness.*

8. Interview with Gerard Desilets in Boston, Massachusetts, 7 June 1984.

9. Robert Alford and Roger Friedland, "Political Participation in Public Policy," *Annual Review of Sociology* 1 (1975):429–479.

10. D. R. Marshall, *The Politics of Participation in Poverty: A Case Study of the Board of Economic and Youth Opportunities Agency of Greater Los Angeles* (Berkeley: University of California Press, 1971).

11. Alford and Friedland, "Political Participation in Public Policy," 447.

12. Starr, *Social Transformation of American Medicine,* 377.

13. Alford and Friedland, "Political Participation," 473.

14. Cyndee Eyster, "Special Report on Health Issues in Election Year '84: State Roundup," *Federation of American Hospitals Review* 17:5 (1984):17–35. According to the FAH, twenty-six states reported they had (or had had) a cost-containment commission operating in their state by 1984. Upon closer scrutiny of the state-by-state report, I discovered that California, Massachusetts, Michigan, and Pennsylvania reported "none," although I had additional information from other sources to contradict these responses. I conclude, therefore, that *at least* thirty states, perhaps more, had established cost-containment commissions of some type by 1984. It is more likely that state reporters would omit the existence of a commission or confuse it with a coalition than report one that had never existed.

15. For further discussions on European styles of corporatism, as well as its application in the American setting, see Leo Panitch, "The Development of Corporatism in Liberal Democracies," in *Trends Toward Corporatist Intermediation,* ed. P. C. Schmitter and G. Lehmbruch (Beverly Hills, Calif.: Sage, 1979); P. C. Schmitter, "Still the Century of Corporatism," *Review of Politics* 36 (1974): 85–131; and Lawrence Brown, "Technocratic Corporatism and Administrative Reform in Medicare," *Journal of Health Politics, Policy and Law* 10:3 (Fall 1985): 579–599.

16. Wolfgang Streeck and P. C. Schmitter, *Private Interest Government, Beyond Market and State* (London: Sage, 1985), vii.

17. R. Seidelman, "Pluralist Heaven's Dissenting Angels: Corporatism in the American Political Economy," in *The Political Economy of Public Policy,* ed. Alan

Stone and Edward Harpham, (Beverly Hills, Calif.: Sage, 1982), 67; James O'Connor, *Accumulation Crisis* (Oxford, England: Basil Blackwell, 1984).

18. Brown, "Technocratic Corporatism," 583.

19. See Alan Cawson, *Corporatism and Political Theory* (New York: Basil Blackwell, 1986),39; and Ross Martin, "Pluralism and the New Corporatism," *Political Studies* 31 (1983):99.

20. See David Easton, *A Systems Analysis of Political Life* (New York: Wiley and Sons, 1965), for a persuasive pluralist description of the state. Other classic explications of pluralism include Robert Dahl, *Who Governs? Power and Democracy in an American City* (New Haven, Conn.: Yale University Press, 1971); David Truman, *The Governmental Process: Political Interests and Public Opinion* (New York: Knopf, 1971); Philip Selznick, *TVA and the Grass Roots* (Berkeley: University of California Press, 1949); and Grant McConnell, *Private Power and American Democracy* (New York: Knopf, 1967). For the most clear defense of corporatism, see Cawson, *Corporatism and Political Theory*.

21. The policy research literature in political science derives from the comparative urban research studies of the 1960s and 1970s that place business power into a model of urban policy-making, in which business participation becomes a "situational" variable in the urban political system, interacting with "structural" and "cultural" variables as they lead to policy decisions. See Robert R. Alford, *Bureaucracy and Participation: Political Culture in Four Wisconsin Cities* (Chicago: Rand McNally, 1969) and Thomas R. Dye, *Politics, Economics and the Public. Policy Outcomes in the American States* (Chicago: Rand McNally, 1966). Business power is measured by political variables such as its degree of decentralization (Terry Clark, "Community Structure, Decision-Making, Budget Expenditures and Renewal in 51 American Communities," *American Sociological Review* 33 [1968]:576–593); organizational differentiation and degree of innovation (Michael Aiken and Robert Alford, "Community Structure and Innovation: The Case of Urban Renewal," *American Sociological Review* 35 [August 1970]:650–665; and Jack Walker "The Diffusion of Innovation Among the American States," *American Political Science Review* 63 [September 1969]:880–900); extralocal linkages (Herman Turk, "Interorganizational Networks in Urban Society: Initial Perspectives and Comparative Research," *American Sociological Review* 35 [February 1970]:1–19); or its economic dominance and mobility (Roger Friedland and Donald Palmer, "Park Place and Main Street: Business and the Urban Power Structure," *Annual Review of Sociology* 10 [1984]:393–416).

Although this book focuses on business as a political independent variable, most research has shown that political variables simply do not explain policy outcomes with the same power as economic ones. Ira Sharkansky and Richard Hofferbert have observed that the measurement of policies and politics by political scientists or political sociologists has been too simple, lacking the necessary precision about dimensions of policy responding to dimensions of politics and economics (Sharkansky and Hofferbert, "Dimensions of State Politics, Economics and Public Policy," *American Political Science Review* 63 [1969]:867–879). However, although political variables have been tested and found to have relatively less direct and independent impact than socioeconomic variables, we should not be too quick to reject the importance of political variables. Only a few type of political variables have been tested in a few contexts, and the results have often been equivocal.

In addition to the study of economic, structural, and political variables in the policy process, a body of policy research studies focuses on the economic and market dominance of business power. These studies address the fundamental relationship of the economic basis of the state to the policy process. See Claus Offe, "The Theory of the Capitalist State and the Problem of Policy Formation," in *Stress and Contradiction in Modern Capitalism* ed. Leon Lindberg et al. (Lexington, Mass.: D.C. Heath, 1975), 125–145; Claus Offe and Volker Ronge, "Theses on the Theory of the State," in *Class, Power and Conflict,* ed. Anthony Giddens and David Held (Berkeley: University of California Press, 1982), 139–147; and James O'Connor, *The Fiscal Crisis of the State* (New York: St. Martins Press, 1973). Specific work on the interaction of capital with the state has also been done by several other authors. See Gabriel Kolko, *The Triumph of Conservatism: A Reinterpretation of American History, 1900–1916* (New York: Free Press, 1967); James Weinstein, *The Corporate Ideal in the Liberal State: 1900–1918* (Boston: Beacon Press, 1968); Schmitter and Lehmbruch, *Trends Towards Corporatist Intermediation;* and Cawson, *Corporatism and Political Theory.* The emphasis in these works has been both the political and economic dominance of representatives of capital in the policy process and the constraints that a capitalist society places on political change. The problem with this research tradition is that too often scholars assume business dominance without proving it.

22.   W. I. Jenkins, *Policy Analysis: A Political and Organisational Perspective* (London: Martin Robertson, 1978), 15. Jenkins's actual definition is "a set of interrelated decisions taken by a political actor or group of actors concerning the selection of goals and the means of achieving them within a specified situation where these decisions should, in principle, be within the power of these actors to achieve."

23.   Joseph T. Nolan, "Political Surfing When the Issues Break," *Harvard Business Review* 63:1 (January–February 1985):73.

24.   Interview with Massachusetts health care coalition participant in Boston, June 1984.

25.   Alford, *Health Care Politics,* 10; see also Herbert Kaufman, "The Political Ingredient of Public Health Services: A Neglected Area of Research," *The Milbank Memorial Fund Quarterly* 44 (October 1966):30–31; Theodore Marmor, *The Politics of Medicare* (Chicago: Aldine Publishing Company, 1973); and Herbert Harvey Hyman, ed. *The Politics of Health Care: Nine Case Studies of Innovative Planning in New York City* (New York: Praeger, 1973).

26.   Marmor, *Politics of Medicare;* and Theodore Marmor, "American Health Politics, 1970 to the Present: Some Comments" (Paper presented at the Health Care Policy Conference, College of William and Mary, Williamsburg, Virginia, November 1987).

27.   For examples of books on health care politics written since the mid-1970s, see Starr, *The Social Transformation of American Medicine;* Alford, *Health Care Politics;* Lawrence Brown, *Politics and Health Care Organization. HMOs as Federal Policy* (Washington, D.C.: Brookings Institution, 1983); Judith Feder, *Medicare: The Politics of Federal Hospital Insurance* (Lexington, Mass.: Lexington Books, 1977); Frank J. Thompson, *Health Policy and the Bureaucracy* (Cam-

bridge, Mass.: MIT Press, 1981); Theodore Marmor, ed. *Political Analysis and American Medical Care* (Cambridge: Cambridge University Press, 1983); and Andrew B. Dunham and James Morone, *The Politics of Innovation: The Evolution of DRG Rate Regulation in New Jersey* (Princeton, N.J.: Health Research and Educational Trust, 1983).

28. Alford, *Health Care Politics*, 14.

29. Havighurst, "The Changing Locus of Decision Making in the Health Care Sector," 697–735.

30. Marc Renaud, "Quebec: The Adventures of a Narcissistic State," in *The End of an Illusion: The Future of Health Policy in Western Industrialized Nations*, ed. J. de Kervasdoue, J. R. Kimberly, and V. Rodwin (Berkeley: University of California Press, 1984).

Chapter Three: Business and the Pushcart Vendors

1. Faltermayer, "Better Care at Less Cost Without Miracles," 127.

2. "It's Time to Operate," *Fortune* (January 1970):79.

3. For a description of foundation interventions in health, see Howard Berliner, "A Larger Perspective on the Flexner Report," *International Journal of Health Services* 5:4 (1975):513–592; and E. R. Brown, *Rockefeller Medicine Men: Medicine and Capitalism in America* (Berkeley: University of California Press, 1979).

4. Funded by eight foundations, the committee was composed of health providers, insurance, and banking representatives. Committee on the Costs of Medical Care, *Medical Care for the American People: The Final Report of the Committee on the Costs of Medical Care* (Chicago: University of Chicago Press, 1932).

5. For a more thorough description of these cycles, see Jack Salmon, "Corporate Attempts to Reorganize the American Health Care System" (Ph.D. diss., Cornell University, 1978), 96–126. For an explanation of economic cycles, see Simon Kuznets, "Long Swings in the Growth of Population and in Related Economic Variables," *Proceedings of the American Philosophical Society* (February 1958): 25–52.

6. See Abraham Flexner, *Medical Education in the United States and Canada*, *Bulletin No. 4* (New York: Carnegie Foundation for the Advancement of Teaching, 1910); and Howard Berliner, *A System of Scientific Medicine: Philanthropic Foundations in the Flexner Era* (New York: Tavistock, 1985).

7. Salmon, "Corporate Attempts to Reorganize," 99. Some background material for this chapter comes from the dissertation of Jack Salmon, currently professor at the University of Illinois at Chicago, whom I thank for his contributions and theoretical framework as well as the rich and extensive bibliography that gave me an excellent review of the literature up to 1978.

8. The material related to business and the insurance industry comes from interviews with Walter McNerney, former president of Blue Cross in Chicago, March 1988, and Bernard Tresnowski, current president of Blue Cross, in Chicago, March 1988. For more information on the development of Blue Cross see Sylvia Law, *Blue Cross: What Went Wrong?* (New Haven, Conn.: Yale University Press, 1974).

9. Interview with McNerney.

10. Salmon, "Corporate Attempts to Reorganize," 120.

11. Useem, *The Inner Circle*, 151.

12. Daniel Holland and Stewart Myers, "Profitability and Capital Costs for Manufacturing Corporations and All Nonfinancial Corporations" *American Economic Review* 70 (1980):320–325. These data are discussed more thoroughly in Useem, *The Inner Circle*, 150–159.

13. A study by Data Resources as quoted in Useem, *The Inner Circle*, 154.

14. Salmon, "Corporate Attempts to Reorganize," 115.

15. "The Big Changes that Reshaped the Decade," *Business Week* (14 September 1974):51–53.

16. John Iglehart, "Health Care and American Business" *The New England Journal of Medicine* 306 (14 January 1982):121.

17. "The Big Changes that Reshaped the Decade," 52.

18. "Special Report: The $60 Billion Crisis Over Medical Care," *Business Week* (17 January 1970):56.

19. Ibid.

20. Demkovich, "Business is Paying Heed to the Bottom Line," 851; Sapolsky, et al., "Corporate Attitudes Toward Health Care Costs," 566; U.S. Chamber of Commerce, "Employee Benefits 1983," *Medical Benefits* 2:4 (28 February 1985):1–3; and "U.S. Industrial Outlook 1989: Health Services," *Medical Benefits* 6:3 (15 February 1989):1–2; Eileen Tell, Marilyn Falik, and Peter Fox, "Private-Sector Health Care Initiatives: A Comparative Perspective from Four Communities," *Milbank Memorial Fund Quarterly/Health and Society* 62:3 (1984):357–379.

21. Louis Uchitelle, "Corporate Profitability Rising, Reversing 15-Year Downturn," *The New York Times* (30 November 1987):1.

22. See Useem, *The Inner Circle*, for a persuasive description of the way in which business elites in the United States and the United Kingdom can influence policy.

23. "It's Time to Operate," *Fortune*, 79.

24. Alford, *Health Care Politics*, 15. Also see Christopher Pollitt, "Corporate Rationalization of American Health Care: A Visitor's Appraisal" *Journal of Health Politics, Policy and Law* 7:1 (Spring 1982):230.

25. Faltermayer, "Better Care at Less Cost Without Miracles," 127.

26. John M. Mecklin, "Hospitals Need Management Even More than Money," *Fortune* (January 1970):96–99.

27. Arnold M. Rose, *The Power Structure, Political Process in American Society* (London: Oxford University Press, 1967), 111.

28. The technique of searching for articles by computer is much faster than the old-fashioned way of looking at microfiche; however, the computer is not as accurate as the old-fashioned human eye, in the sense that some articles may contain the key words but not really fit the definition of relevance, while other articles that deal directly with the topic may not show up in the search at all. Although I have screened these articles for relevancy, these data should only be interpreted as suggestive of general trends, not as proof of actual numbers of articles on the topic. The years 1969–1971 are not included because *Fortune* and *Forbes* did not start their database until September 1971 and *Business Week* did not begin

until November 1972. Therefore, there are probably more relevant articles in 1972–1973 than the table indicates.

29. Useem, *The Inner Circle,* 89–90.

30. Week, "The $60 Billion Crisis," 56.

31. Ibid., 64.

32. Some examples of the articles include J. S. Lublin, "Seeking a Cure: Companies Fight Back Against Soaring Costs of Medical Coverage," *Wall Street Journal* (10 May 1978):1; "Editorial: A Place for HMOs," *Business Week* (12 January 1974):80; H. Schwartz, "R. J. Reynolds Takes the Hippocratic Oath," *New York Times* (7 August 1977): section 1:1.

33. Committee on the Costs of Medical Care, *Medical Care for the American People.*

34. Ibid., 90.

35. Irving Shapiro, *America's Third Revolution: Public Interest and the Private Role* (New York: Harper & Row, 1984).

36. See Council on Wage and Price Stability, *The Problem of Rising Health Care Costs* (Washington, D.C.: U.S. Government Printing Office, 26 April 1976), and *The Complex Puzzle of Rising Health Care Costs: Can the Private Sector Fit it Together?* (Washington, D.C.: U.S. Government Printing Office, December 1976), ii–iii.

37. Other articles addressing this issue include: "Ford to Start Own HMO," *Wall Street Journal* (10 May 1978); "Containing the Costs of Employee Health Plans," *Business Week* (30 May 1977); Lublin, "Seeking a Cure," 1.

38. Robert Pear, "Companies Tackle Health Care Costs," *New York Times* (Sunday, 3 March 1985):section F, 11.

39. Graham Wilson, *Business and Politics* 130.

Chapter Four: Institutional Mechanisms for Change

1. President of the Washington Business Group on Health, Washington, D.C. All quoted material in this chapter attributed to Goldbeck, if not cited in a published article, comes from taped interviews by this author with Goldbeck in April, June, and November 1984 in Washington, D.C.

2. Shapiro, *America's Third Revolution;* Dunlop, *Business and Public Policy;* Domhoff, *The Higher Circles* and *The Powers That Be.*

3. Sar A. Levitan and Martha Cooper, *Business Lobbies: The Public Good and the Bottom Line* (Baltimore: Johns Hopkins University Press, 1984).

4. Kirkland, "Fat Days for the Chamber of Commerce," 145–157.

5. Interview with Jan Ozga, health policy staff to the U.S. Chamber of Commerce, Washington, D.C., 18 June 1984.

Provider conflict can be partially explained by the Chamber's membership. The newest health member of the Chamber in 1983 was James Sammons of the AMA. Other provider members included representatives of the AHA, Hospital Corporation of America (HCA, a for-profit hospital corporation), and Eli Lilly and Company, a drug manufacturer. Business conflict came over the dominance of insurer members on Chamber committees, particularly when insurer members promoted regulatory health policy solutions contrary to solutions being promoted by the Reagan administration.

6.   Telephone interview with Willis Goldbeck, WBGH, Washington, D.C., 18 November 1984.

7.   Interview with David Winston, then vice president of strategy for Voluntary Hospitals of America in Washington, D.C., 29 November 1984. All quotes in this chapter attributed to Winston are from this interview. Due to a fatal accident in 1986, David Winston was never able to verify his point of view for this book; however, I had tape recorded the two hour interview with him.

8.   Note the way in which elite groups in control of policy will attempt to resolve conflict among other elites. Winston and the White House used the countervailing power of purchasers and other provider interests to balance the perceived domination by insurers of the health policy process at the Chamber.

9.   Clearinghouse on Business Coalitions for Health Action, "Directory of Business Coalitions for Health Action" (April 1984), i; Peter A. Holmes, "Competition Comes to Medical Care," *Nation's Business* (April 1984):18.

10.   Peter Slavin, "The Business Roundtable: New Lobbying Arm of Big Business," *Business and Society Review* (Winter 1975 to 1976):28–32.

11.   Domhoff, *The Powers That Be*, 79.

12.   Interview with a vice president of TRW in Washington, D.C., June 1984.

13.   Interview with an AHA staff member, Chicago, March 1988.

14.   Interview with Frederick Lee, director of public policy issues, WBGH, Washington, D.C. December 1984.

15.   Basic information on the way in which the Roundtable dealt with health policy comes from two main sources: interviews with John T. Dunlop of Harvard University, in Cambridge, Mass., 18 May 1987 and 10 September 1987; and a telephone interview with Nicholas La Trenta, a vice president with Metropolitan Life Insurance Company, who was staff to John Creedon on the Dunlop Group and staff to the Roundtable's Health Care Task Force when Creedon was chair, 11 December 1987.

16.   Business Roundtable, "An Appropriate Role for Corporations in Health Care Cost Management," February 1982, 1–9.

17.   Linda Demkovich, "On Health Issues, This Business Group is a Leader, but is Anyone Following?" *National Journal* (18 June 1983):1278.

18.   Willis Goldbeck, "Health and Work in America: A Brief Look into the 21st Century" (Presentation at the Pew Health Policy Fellows conference, Boston, Mass., May 1987).

19.   American Hospital Association, "1986–1987 Survey of Health Care Coalitions," *Medical Benefits* (30 September 1987):4.

20.   These states included Illinois, Iowa, Pennsylvania, and Colorado, among others. California was one of several states that killed their state data agency in the early 1980s in a flush of so-called "competitive, antiregulatory" sentiment, much to the dismay of the business coalitions in the state, who helped salvage the data function by moving its management to the State Department of Health.

21.   Alford and Friedland, "Political Participation and Public Policy."

22.   Because almost nothing is written on the proceedings of the Dunlop Group, information on the Dunlop Group comes from various sources, including inter-

views, books, and articles. Interviews were conducted with Dunlop himself on three different occasions in Cambridge, Mass., in 1987. I also conducted interviews in 1987 and 1988 with Galen Young of the AHA, chief staff to Dunlop for meetings: Bernard Tresnowski, president of Blue Cross and Blue Shield, and Walter McNerney, former president of Blue Cross; Jim Sammons, executive vice president of the AMA; Alexander Williams, vice president of the AHA; Nicholas La Trenta, of Metropolitan Life; and Bert Seidman, director of the Department of Occupational Safety, Health and Social Security of the AFL-CIO. Interviews were attempted with Carl Schramm, current president of the HIAA, and Carol McCarthy, president of the AHA, but neither would agree to be interviewed.

23. American Hospital Association, "Digest of National Health Care Use and Expense Indicators," December 1986.

24. Samuel Huntington, *American Politics: The Promise of Disharmony* (Cambridge, Mass.: Belknap Press, 1981).

25. John T. Dunlop, *Private Sector Coalitions: A Fourth Party in Health Care?*, ed. Jon Jaeger (Durham, N.C.: Duke University Press, 1983), 8; and Clark Havighurst, *Private-Sector Coalitions*, 44.

26. Clearinghouse on Business Coalitions for Health Action, "Directory of Business Coalitions for Health Action" (Washington: Chamber of Commerce of the U.S. 1982). The numbers for 1983 and 1985 come from the AHA's surveys of health care coalitions for those years; the 1987 number comes from an evaluation of the AHA's data bank by Lawrence Brown and Catherine McLaughlin, conducted in 1987.

27. A sample of the many articles and books on coalitions includes the following: Jon Jaeger, ed., *Private Sector Coalitions: A Fourth Party in Health Care?*; Government Research Corporation, *A Report on Coalitions to Contain Health Care Costs* (Washington, D.C.: Government Research Corporation, 1979); Willis Goldbeck, "Health Care Coalitions," in *Health Care Cost Management*, ed. Peter D. Fox, Willis B. Goldbeck, and Jacob J. Spies, (Ann Arbor, Mich.: Health Administration Press, 1984); Jane Stein, "New Goals for Business Coalitions," *Business and Health* 2:7 (June 1985):42–45; Allen Meyerhoff and David A. Crozier, "Health Care Coalitions: The Evolution of a Movement," *Health Affairs* 3:1 (Spring 1984):120–129; Lawrence D. Brown and Catherine G. McLaughlin, " 'May the Third Force Be With You': Community Programs for Affordable Health Care," in *Advances in Health Economics and Health Services Research, Vol. 8*, ed. Richard Scheffler and L. F. Rossiter (Greenwich, Conn.; JAI Press, 1988); Joyce Lanning and Myron D. Fottler, "Coalitions for Health Care: New Interorganizational Relations Affecting the Delivery of Health Care" (Paper, January 1984); Paul Gerber, "How Health Care Coalitions Will Affect Your Practice," *Physician's Management* (February 1986):200–215; Symond Gottlieb, "Ensuring Access to Health Care: What Communities Can Do to Make a Difference Through Private Sector Coalitions," *Inquiry* 23 (Fall 1986):322–329; Irwin Miller, "Interpreneurship: A Community Coalition Approach to Health Care Reform," *Inquiry* 24 (Fall 1987):266–275; Chris York, "Business and 'the Common'," *Inquiry* 23 (Fall 1986):299–307; and Linda Bergthold, "Crabs in a Bucket: The Politics of Health Care Reform in California," *Journal of Health Politics, Policy and Law* 9:2 (Summer 1984):203–222; and Bergthold, "Purchasing

Power: Business and Health Policy Change in Massachusetts," *Journal of Health Politics, Policy and Law* 13:3 (Fall 1988):425–451. Sources for these terms are: "third force"—Lawrence Brown and Catherine McLaughlin; "fourth party"—a consortium of interested parties who participated in a forum resulting in *Private Sector Coalitions: A Fourth Party in Health Care?*; "buyers cartels"—Alexander Williams of the AHA; "countervailing force"—John K. Galbraith, who used the term to describe a strong buyer that offsets a strong seller, and Robert Alford, who reinterpreted the term to apply to health care in *Health Care Politics*.

28.   Lanning and Fottler, "Coalitions for Health Care"; and AMA spokesman, as quoted in Jaeger, ed., *Private Sector Coalitions*, 17.

29.   Ibid., 44.

30.   Ibid., 11.

31.   A few years after the Dunlop Group began meeting, the Robert Wood Johnson Foundation initiated its program on "Community Programs for Affordable Health Care," a program that Dunlop and his cohorts helped to structure and implement and that would ultimately result in the commitment of about $20 million to the stimulation and development of sixteen community health care coalitions that imitated the Dunlop Group composition, although more than three hundred groups applied. (See Jaeger, ed., *Private Sector Coalitions*.)

32.   Galen Wilsey Young, "Coalitions are Defined, Data Base Described by AHA's Office of Health Care Coalitions," *Health Care Vigil* (15 April 1983):1.

33.   Goldbeck, "Health Care Coalitions," 2.

34.   Clearinghouse on Business Coalitions for Health Action (March 1983):iii.

35.   Telephone interview with one of the Robert Wood Johnson evaluators, Catherine McLaughlin, March 1988.

36.   Stein, "New Goals for Business Coalitions," 45.

37.   Chris York, *Private Sector Coalitions*, 41.

38.   David Rosenbaum, "Chrysler, Hit Hard by Costs, Studies Health Care System," *New York Times* (4 March 1984):10.

39.   Paul Gerber, "How Health Care Coalitions Will Affect Your Practice," 202.

40.   Terence Johnson, *Professions and Power* (London: Macmillan, 1972), 59. For further elaboration on the clashes between expert and managerial autonomy in medicine see Starr, *The Social Transformation of American Medicine*; Charles Perrow, *Complex Organizations* (New York: Random House, 1979); Magali Sarfatti Larson, *The Rise of Professionalism* (Berkeley: University of California Press, 1977).

41.   "It's High Noon in Arizona for Hospital Costs," *Business Week* (13 February 1984):43.

42.   John K. Iglehart, "Big Business and Health Care in the Heartland," 43.

43.   "Leaders Debate Effectiveness of Groups," *Benefits Today* (31 July 1987): 259.

44.   Steven L. Seiler, "The Management Perspective on Coalitions," in Jon Jaeger, ed., *Private Sector Coalitions*, 21.

45.   Seymour M. Lipset, *Political Man: The Social Bases of Politics* (Baltimore, Md.: Johns Hopkins University Press, 1981); Huntington, *American Politics*, 110.

46.   Miller, "Interpreneurship," 270.

47.   Louis Harris and Associates, Inc. "The Equitable Healthcare Survey, Options for Controlling Costs," Equitable Life Assurance Society, August 1983.
48.   Business Roundtable Task Force on Health, "Corporate Health Care Cost Management and Private Sector Initiatives, 1984 Survey."
49.   American Hospital Association, "1986–1987 Survey of Health Care Coalitions."
50.   Meyerhoff and Crozier, "Health Care Coalitions," 120–127; and Brown and McLaughlin, " 'May the Third Force Be With You.' "
51.   "Leaders Debate Effectiveness of Groups," 259.
52.   Brown and McLaughlin, " 'May the Third Force Be With You,' " 18.
53.   Ibid., 35.

Chapter Five: The Federal Context: A Wedge of Structural Change

1.   Stephen Cohen and Charles Goldfinger, "From Permacrisis to Real Crisis in French Social Security: The Limits to Normal Politics," in *Stress and Contradiction in Modern Capitalism*, ed. Leon Lindberg et al. (Lexington, Mass: D.C. Heath, 1975), 91.
2.   Lawrence D. Brown, "Washington Report," *Journal of Health Politics, Policy and Law* 6:4 (Winter 1982):822–826.
3.   Robert Evans, "Finding the Levers, Finding the Courage: Lessons from Cost Containment in North America," *Journal of Health Politics, Policy and Law* 11:4 (1986):610.
4.   Havighurst, "The Changing Locus of Decision Making in the Health Care Sector," 723.
5.   The Walsh Group was chaired by William Walsh, M.D., a founder of Project HOPE, a think tank in Millwood, Virginia, and friend and adviser of Ronald Reagan. Memorandum to William J. Casey, Edwin W. Meese, Martin C. Anderson, from William B. Walsh, M.D., chairman, health policy advisory group to President-elect Reagan, pp. 1–20.

Members of the Walsh Health Policy Advisory Group included: William Walsh, chairman—president and medical director, the People-to-People Health Foundation, Inc. (Project HOPE); Rita Ricardo-Campbell, senior fellow, the Hoover Institute and American Enterprise Institute; James Cavanagh, senior vice president, Allergan Pharmaceutical Company, former deputy chief of staff at the White House, former deputy director of the Domestic Council, and former deputy assistant secretary of HEW; Theodore Cooper, executive vice president of the Upjohn pharmaceutical company, former dean of Cornell University Medical College, and former assistant secretary of HEW for health; Dr. Charles Edwards, president, Scripps Clinic and Research foundation, former assistant secretary of HEW for health, and former commissioner of the Food and Drug Administration; Isaac Ehrlich, professor of Economics, State University of New York, Buffalo; Alain Enthoven, professor of public and private management, Stanford University Graduate School of Business; Dr. William Felch, former chairman of AMA legislative council; Clark Havighurst, professor, Duke University School of Law and former professor of community health sciences, Duke University Medical

School; Helen Jameson, assistant administrator, Rochester Methodist University; Cotton Lindsay, visiting professor of economics, Emory University; William Longmire, Jr., professor of surgery, University of California at Los Angeles School of Medicine, and former president of American College of Surgeons; Wade Mountz, former chairman, legislative council, American Hospital Association; Mary Runge, chair of the board, American Pharmaceutical Association; Lee Shelton, director of health services, Health First, Atlanta, Georgia, and former member, FDA National Advisory Committee on Drugs; Robert Shira, senior vice president and acting provost, Tufts University, and former president, American Dental Association; C. Joseph Stetler, former president, American Pharmaceutical Manufacturers Association; Frank Stinchfield, practicing surgeon at Columbia Presbyterian Medical Center and former president, American College of Surgeons. "Medicine and Health," 34:44 (10 November 1980):8.

6.   John Iglehart, "Drawing the Lines for the Debate on Competition," *The New England Journal of Medicine* 305:5 (30 July, 1981):292.

7.   Walsh memo, 4.

8.   The Winston task force was officially called the "Private Sector Task Force on Competition." Its members included: Chairman David A. Winston, senior vice president with Blyth Eastman Paine Webber, Health Care Funding, Inc., former staff to the California Assembly under Governor Reagan, and former staff to Sen. Richard Schweiker; Jack Anderson, president, Manor Care, Inc.; Karl Bays, chairman and CEO, American Hospital Supply Corporation; Michael Bromberg, director, Federation of American Hospitals; Dr. Claire Fagin, dean, School of Nursing, University of Pennsylvania; Max W. Fine, president, Health Cost Management Systems, Inc.; Clark Havighurst, professor, Duke University School of Law; John F. Horty, president, National Council of Community Hospitals; John Kittredge, executive vice president, Prudential Insurance Company; Bernard Lachner, Evanston Hospital, Illinois; David Main, lawyer, Epstein Becker Borsody and Green; Walter McNerney, president, Blue Cross Association; Thomas Nesbitt, M.D., Urology Associations, Nashville Tennessee; Uwe Reinhardt, professor, Woodrow Wilson School, Princeton University; Dr. William Rial, president, AMA; Jack Shelton, manager, Employee Insurance Department, Ford Motor Company; C. Joseph Stetler, Dickstein, Shapiro, and Morin and former president of Pharmaceutical Manufacturers Association; Nathan Tannern, McKay-Dee Hospital Center, a volunteer trustee of the not-for-profit hospitals; Samuel Tibbitts, president, Lutheran Hospital Society, James A. Vohs, president and chairman of the board, Kaiser Foundation Health Plan; William Walsh, M.D., Project HOPE; James Whitman, president, Hospital Financial Management Association; and Christopher York, vice president, Citibank N.A. Note: Both business representatives came from the second echelon of elite power; neither was a CEO. Their CEO counterparts, whom Winston would have liked to join the task force, would have been Henry Ford, Jr., and Walter Wriston; both were prominent founding members of the Business Roundtable.

9.   "Task Force Report on Competition Legislation," December 1981, submitted by the Private Sector Task Force on Competition Chairman David Winston.

10.   Linda Demkovich, "States May Be Gaining in the Battle to Curb Medicaid Spending Growth," *National Journal* 14:38 (18 September 1982):1584.

11.   Levitan and Cooper, *Business Lobbies*, 112.

12.   The information on the Winston task force and the White House efforts to push through their program comes from articles and interviews with knowledgeable Washington policy observers, including David Winston.

13.   In the passage of California's 1982 MediCal Reform, the state created an office directed by William Guy, formerly with Blue Cross, to conduct the state contract negotiations with hospitals. The press quickly dubbed Guy the "czar," a term that reflected the independence and aggressive stance of his office. See Chapter 6 for a more detailed description of the California reforms.

14.   Medicare had traditionally reimbursed hospitals on an implicit per diem system, where hospitals could charge Medicare by the day; the new system was a radical shift from that mechanism to a per case system of payment. Medicare would now pay hospitals by the type of the illness, not the number of days it took to cure and discharge the patient. Costs higher than 120 percent of the average costs of comparable hospitals would no longer be considered "reasonable costs." The hospitals would receive some adjustment for "outlier" patients and for area wages. Otherwise, no adjustment was to be made for the severity of the illness. Judith Lave, "Hospital Payment Under Medicare," as quoted from the "Conference on the Future of Medicare," Committee on Ways and Means, U.S. House of Representatives, 29 November 1983.

15.   The state of Arizona was considered a backslider by the Reagan loyalists because it distorted the mandate of new Federalism. Four large corporations in Arizona tried to get health care reform through the legislature in 1983 and 1984; failing to get the bill that business wanted, the business coalitions formed by these corporations collected signatures and placed three initiatives on the ballot. All of this would have been considered fine with the new Federalists, except that business chose to propose the regulation of the health care system and rejected a competitive solution.

16.   Demkovich, "States May Be Gaining," 1584.

17.   As quoted to me in an interview in December 1984, 75 percent of the savings achieved by the Bank of America in California in the cost of health care premiums for their employees was from a cost shift to employees. Robert Pear cites similar statistics in *The New York Times* (Sunday, 2 March 1985):section F, 11.

Chapter Six: Crabs in a Bucket: Business and Health Policy Change in California

1.   Meeting of the Santa Cruz Medical Society, Aptos Seascape Lodge, Santa Cruz, California, 8 February 1983.

2.   The MediCal reform legislation of 1982 included several structural changes, program reductions, and other cost-containment measures. The structural changes included: (1) a special negotiator who would contract for the state of California, through either bidding or negotiation, with various providers of institutional and noninstitutional services for Medicaid beneficiaries; (2) contracting for services with noninstitutional providers to provide case management for beneficiaries by the Department of Health Services; (3) authorization for Blue

Cross and commercial insurers to contract with institutional and professional providers for reduced rates for group policyholders who chose participating providers; (4) elimination of the Medically Indigent Adult program from state responsibility (larger counties would receive a block grant of approximately 70 percent of previous funding levels from the state and could design their own program for MIAs; smaller counties were offered the same option); (5) consolidation of Short-Doyle and MediCal mental health services. Program reductions included: (1) benefit reductions (services such a podiatric, rehabilitation therapies, adult vision care, eyeglasses, and nonemergency transportation would need provider's justification that the service was necessary to protect life or prevent significant disability; (2) eligibility changes that made it more difficult for potential beneficiaries to qualify for service; (3) reimbursement reductions of 10 percent for services such as physician and outpatient, acupuncture, chiropractic, and psychological services. Other cost-containment measures included: (1) authorization for the Department of Health Services to enter into contracts for volume purchasing of drugs, appliances, lab, and other health care products; (2) a reduction in funds for teaching hospitals at the University of California; (3) improvements in audit procedures. This summary is extracted from Leonard Aucoin and Leonard Duhl, M.D., "The 1982 California Health Care Reform: A Case Study in Policy Analysis," Paper prepared for Western Consortium for the Health Professions, San Francisco, January 1983, 33–40.

3.   This coalition was organized as the Roberti Cost Containment Commission, but the broader definition of the coalition includes almost a dozen employer or business coalitions thoroughout the state that also participated in the passage of this legislation. The 1982 Roberti Coalition members included: twelve members of business, representing general business interests and business coalitions— San Diego Employers' Health Cost Coalition, The California Council of Health Care Coalitions, The Employers' Health Care Coalition of Los Angeles, Inland Employers' Health Coalition, Industrial Relations Task Force of Santa Clara County, Diablo Valley Coalition, Health Care Roundtable of Greater Sacramento, Subcommittee on Health Legislation of the California Chamber of Commerce, Orange County Employers' Health Care Coalition, Alameda County Employers Coalition, and Fresno Coalition. Labor had twelve members, representing the United Steelworkers of America, Board of Carpenters, United Auto Workers, Service Employees International Union, Transportation Union, Teamsters, Machinists, Longshoremen, Operating Engineers, Communication Workers (two unions, California State Employees Association and California School Employees Association, were added in 1983).

Senior Citizens had seven members, including representatives of the Commission on Aging, the Retired Teachers Association, American Association of Retired Persons, Congress of Senior Citizens, Gray Panthers, and National Association of Retired Federal Employees. In the 1982 Roberti Coalition hospitals and the medical association were also represented; in 1983 they were removed and placed on an "expert," nonvoting task force of thirty-four members.

4.   Ed Salzman, "Has California Launched a National Health Care Revolution?" *California Journal* 13:8 (August 1982): 290–292.

5.   See n. 12 below for clarification of market and regulatory or bureaucratic reforms.

6.   Presentation by Dr. Leonard J. Duhl at a conference in Monterey, California, 2 November 1982. For additional comments on California's MediCal Reform, see E. P. Melia, L. M. Aucoin, L. J. Duhl, and P. S. Kurokawa, "Competition in the Healthcare Marketplace: A Beginning in California," *New England Journal of Medicine* 308 (31 March, 1983):788–92.

7.   Dr. Philip Lee, director of the Institute for Health Policy Studies, University of California at San Francisco (Presentation, conference on the medically indigent adult, Santa Cruz, Calif., 2 December 1982).

8.   "Analysis of the Budget Bill of the State of California for the Fiscal Year July 1, 1982, to June 30, 1983"; "Report of the Legislative Analyst to the Joint Legislative Budget Committee" (Sacramento; State of California, 24 February 1982).

9.   Charlene Harrington et al., "California: State Discretionary Policies and Services in the Medicaid, Social Services and Supplementary Security Income Programs" (San Francisco: Aging Health Policy Center, UCSF, 1982), 8–11. MIAs are adults under sixty-five who are not eligible for public assistance or as medically needy because they do not meet the requirements that would link them to those federal/state categories. When they become ill, their income is too low to pay for the high costs of medical care, and they become eligible to be MIAs. The cost of this MediCal category was the responsibility of the state of California until 1982 when the MIA program was eliminated from state responsibility by this legislation.

10.   Several articles refer to California's experience with contracting or designing alternative delivery systems for the poor; see California Department of Health, "Prepaid Health Plans: The California Experience," in U.S. Congress, Senate Committee on Government Operations, Permanent Subcommittee on Investigations, *Prepaid Health Plans, Hearings*, 94th Cong., 1st sess. 13–14 March 1975; David F. Chavkin and Anne Treseder, "California's Prepaid Health Plan Program: Can the Patient be Saved?" *Hastings Law Journal* 28 (January 1977):685–760; Victor P. Goldberg, "Some Emerging Problems of Prepaid Health Plans in the MediCal System," *Policy Analysis* 1:1 (Winter 1975):55–68; and Bruce Spitz, "When a Solution is Not a Solution: Medicaid and Health Maintenance Organizations," *Journal of Health Politics, Policy and Law* 3:4 (Winter 1979):497–518.

11.   "Analysis of the Budget Bill of California."

12.   Generally in this case, market will be used equivalently with competitive when referring to styles of policy change. These terms will be interpreted loosely to mean an approach to cost containment that relies more on the economic forces of the marketplace of medical care and less on regulations promulgated by state bureaucracy. Regulation will be used most often to refer to rate setting, a type of cost containment where a state or other central agency sets hospital rates under some uniform set of criteria. In spite of these distinctions, the difference between these terms is clearly one of degree.

13.   Telephone interview with William Guy, the MediCal "czar or special negotiator," 17 February 1983.

14.   Aucoin and Duhl, "The 1982 California Health Care Reform," 33–40.

15.   Of hospitals in California 43 percent are investor-owned. California has a larger number of investor-owned hospitals than any other state; *California Hospital Factbook* (Sacramento: California Hospital Association Publication, 1981).

"Thirty-four of the nation's 203 HMOs are in California. In August 1978, California had 47.5% of the nation's HMO enrollees." From Lewis Butler et al., "Medical Life on the Western Frontier: The Competitive Impact of Prepaid Medical Care Plans in California" (Berkeley: Institute for Government Studies, 1980), 4.

16.   "Health Outline" (Sacramento: California Assembly Office of Research, no date), 16.

17.   Interview with Gordon Rude, staff to the senate research committee and one architect of the Roberti Coalition strategy, in Sacramento, 14 June 1983.

18.   "First Reading: A Report on Government Affairs" 2:9 (California Hospital Association, 21 April 1982). In this article entitled "Behind Closed Doors," the CHA strongly criticizes the secret, behind-the-scenes discussion by the legislators. Members of the Wednesday Group included Governor Brown (D), Assembly Speaker Willie Brown (D), Senate President Pro Tem David Roberti (D), Senate Majority Floor Leader John Garamendi (D), Assembly Majority Caucus Chairman Richard Robinson (D), Assemblyman Charles Imbrecht (R), Assembly Minority Floor Leader Robert Naylor (R), Assemblyman Richard Mountjoy (R), Senate Minority Caucus Chairman Ken Maddy (R), Senator Bob Beverly (R), and Senator William Campbell (R). According to the legislative staff, the introduction of several different bills at the same time was not a strategic choice but simply a coincidence.

19.   Interview with Dennis Flatt, chief of staff to Senator Garamendi, Sacramento, 12 November 1982.

20.   See n. 3 above for a complete list of participants in the 1982 and 1983 Roberti Coalitions.

21.   Interview with Gordon Rude, 14 June 1983.

22.   Information contained in a letter sent to all members of the California State Legislature by the California Chamber of Commerce on 28 April 1982. See also, "Hospital Cost-Shifting: The Hidden Tax," a HIAA publication (1981).

23.   Interview with Pat Chase, by Dr. Jerry Briscoe of the University of the Pacific, Stockton, California, on 6 October 1982, in Sacramento. Chase was an aide to Senator Roberti and staff to the Roberti Coalition. I wish to express my gratitude to Dr. Briscoe for sharing his interview notes. Without his notes, this research would not have been as detailed or complete.

24.   See Table 8.1 for a breakdown of the business membership in the San Francisco Business Coalition and the Roberti Coalition.

25.   Interview with Bob Lee, vice president of Plantronics, past chairman of the Health Care Cost Containment Committee of the Santa Clara Manufacturing Group, and a member of the Roberti Coalition, San Jose, 18 March 1983.

26.   "CMA News," 29 January 1982.

27.   Interview with Nancy Sullivan of the California Chamber of Commerce at the Santa Clara Manufacturing Group conference on health care cost containment, 18 March 1983; follow-up telephone interview in July 1983.

28.   Letters from the California Manufacturing Association and the California Taxpayers Association to state legislators on 28 April 1982.

29.   "CMA News," 29 January 1982.

30.   Ibid.; this was the first of several instances where the CMA ended up snapping at the heels of the wrong issue.

31. "CMA News," 4 June 1982.

32. Gordon R. Cumming, "What Will Be the Picture of Hospital Services for 1990?" Reprinted by the California Health Facilities Commission, 31 July 1980.

33. Interview with Bill Moseley, legislative aide to the Assembly Republicans, by Dr. Briscoe on 8 November 1982; Bill Moseley (Presentation, conference on the medically indigent adult, Santa Cruz, 2 December 1982).

34. Interview with Dr. Charles White, vice president of research for the California Hospital Association, at Dominican Santa Cruz Hospital, 5 November 1982.

35. Interview by Dr. Briscoe with Lew Keller of the ACLIC, 28 October 1982.

36. Butler et al., "Medical Life on the Western Frontier," 7.

37. "First Reading," a CHA newsletter, 2 June 1982.

The insurers' policy statement is quoted in the CHA newsletter: "There is no prohibition against such private contracts now, but hospitals have shown no willingness to negotiate them and the present market provides little motivation for them to do so. We believe that when prospective MediCal hospital contracts are implemented, the cost shift will eventually be accentuated. We are asking that the Legislature make a change in the health insurance law that will encourage such contracts without statutory compulsion. Present law compels insurance companies to accord policy-holders free choice of physicians and hospitals. We believe that provision is no longer necessary or appropriate. . . . We urge you to give the private carriers some assistance . . . by repealing the last paragraph of Section 10133 and Section 11512 (h) of the Insurance Code."

38. Jim Lewis, "Proposition 13 for Health Costs: How the Health Revolution Will Affect Most Californians," *California Journal* 13:11 (November 1982): 403–405.

39. See report by Lucy Johns, "Some Preliminary Findings from the Hartford-NGA Study," based on work performed on the project, "Changes in Hospital Reimbursement in California: An Analysis of History, Impact and Policy Issues" (Presentation, UC Extension Conference, 14 July 1983), 2. Ms. Johns concludes about this reform process: "forces created the MediCal crisis—leadership got the state out it".

40. Telephone interview with William Guy, 17 February 1983.

41. Briscoe interview with Lew Keller and with Emory "Soap" Dowell of Blue Cross, 7 September 1982.

42. News headlines from the *Sacramento Bee* (1 September 1982) and the *California Journal* (November 1982).

43. Interview with Dr. Charles White, 5 November 1982.

44. "First Reading," a CHA Newsletter, 26 July 1982.

45. "CMA News," 1 October 1982. The actual wording in the newsletter reported "concessions" in several areas: (1) quality assurance—CMA got the legislature to include oversight by "professionally recognized unrelated third parties"; (2) protection for physicians from pressure by hospitals; (3) tried to get the prepaid health plans contracting put under the Knox-Keene Act but failed; (4) eliminated the "middle man" in the insurance contracting, making the contractor the insurer itself; (5) amended the open-staffing provision to allow exclusive contracts for anaesthesiology, pathology, and radiology only; and (6) put off date of contracting from January to July 1983.

46.   Advice given to local physicians by the president of the Santa Cruz Medical Society at their monthly meeting, 8 February 1983.

47.   Santa Clara Manufacturing Group, Documents (Cost-Containment Conference, San Jose, Calif., 18 March 1983).

48.   Interview with Steve Thompson, chief of staff to Speaker Willie Brown, Sacramento, 23 November 1982. Risk capitation describes prepayment for patients based on a fixed amount of money for care, paid in advance to the institution giving that care. The risk involved is placed on the providers of care not to exceed budgeted costs.

49.   Governor Jerry Brown, as quoted in Jim Lewis, "Historic MediCal Legislation," *Sacramento Bee* (27 June 1982):1.

50.   Telephone interview with Hellan Dowden, lobbyist for SEIU and member of the Roberti Coalition representing SEIU, 17 March 1983.

51.   These figures were quoted in 1983 to a member of the Health Care Cost Containment Committee of the Santa Clara Manufacturing Group by the president of the CMA.

52.   From an unpublished paper based on interviews conducted by Dr. Jerry Briscoe, 1983.

53.   U.S. Chamber of Commerce, *Directory of Business Coalitions*, 1984, and Dunlop Group of Six, *Survey of Business Coalitions*, 1986.

54.   For discussion of Michigan experience, see Pamela Paul-Shaheen and Eugenia S. Carpenter, "Legislating Hospital Bed Reduction: The Michigan Experience," *Journal of Health Politics, Policy and Law* 6:4 (Winter 1982):653–675.

55.   John Jacobs, "Battling Health Care Cost Spiral," *San Francisco Sunday Examiner and Chronicle* (7 March 1982):64. Also see Jim Lewis, "Proposition 13 for Medical Costs," 403–405.

56.   In an interview with Gordon Rude, staff to the Roberti Coalition, this author specifically asked how business had been influential in the legislative process. Was it through contributions, through specific contacts? Rude replied that although business members did participate in those ways, the notion of business support more likely brought around the Republicans and impressed the Democrats.

57.   Lewis, "How the Health Revolution Will Affect Most Californians."

58.   Paul Starr, "The Triumph of Accommodation," *Journal of Health Politics, Policy and Law* 7:2 (Fall 1982):622.

59.   Interview with Sen. John Garamendi in *The San Jose Mercury News* (19 March 1983):11B.

60.   Starr, *The Social Transformation of American Medicine*, 333.

61.   As quoted by Hellan Dowden of the SEIU in an interview, 17 March 1983.

62.   Emily Friedman, "MediCal Contracting: Model or Mayhem?" *Hospitals* 58:15 (1, August 1984):74–78.

63.   Robert Lindsey, "Changes in Paying for Health Care Reduce Costs in California, Officials Say," *The New York Times* (Sunday, 20 November 1983):30.

64.   Christopher Bellavita, "California's Health Policy Reform and the Poor," *Public Affairs Report* 24:5 (Berkeley: Institute of Governmental Studies, October 1983):1–8.

65.   Nicole Lurie et al., "Termination from MediCal—Does it Affect Health,"

New   England   Journal   of   Medicine   311:7   (16   August   1984):
480–484.
66.   Friedman, "MediCal Contracting," 76.
67.   Erica Goode, "Hospital Costs Slowing," *The San Francisco Chronicle* (21
February 1985):1.

Chapter Seven: Purchasing Power, Business, and Health Policy
Change in Massachusetts

1.   Commonwealth of Massachusetts, August 10, 1982, *Chapter 372: An Act
Related to Establishment of Hospital Rates of Payment and Charges*, an amendment to Chapter 6A of the General Laws, Section 58.
2.   Valerie Jacoby, "Chapter 372: Its Antecedents, Payment Methodology,
and Legal Implications for Medicaid Patients" Paper, Harvard School of Public
Health Seminar, Cambridge, Mass., May 28, 1983.
3.   For more discussion on this topic, see Cawson, *Corporatism and Political
Theory*; McConnell, *Private Power and American Democracy*; Andrew Shonfield, *Modern Capitalism: The Changing Balance of Public and Private Power*
(New York: Oxford University Press, 1969); and L. Panitch, "The Development
of Corporatism in Liberal Democracies."
4.   McConnell, *Private Power and American Democracy*, 163–164.
5.   Charlene Harrington, "Comparative Study of Long Term Care in Eight
States," Draft report (San Francisco: Aging Health Policy Center, University of
California, 20, December 1983), 4–9.
6.   Massachusetts Business Roundtable, *Health Care Costs in Massachusetts:
A Report of the Health Care Task Force* (May 1982), 1–2.
7.   Alan Sager, "Changes in Financing Uncompensated Hospital Care in Massachusetts, 1982–1987: Motives, Mechanics and Meanings for Access," (Paper,
Boston University School of Public Health, Boston, Mass. 1987), 59.
8.   Boston Urban Study Group, *Who Rules Boston?: A Citizen's Guide to Re-
claiming the City* (Boston, Mass.: Institute for Democratic Socialism, 1984), 25.
9.   Interview with Benjamin Katcoff, vice president of personnel, Polaroid Corporation, Cambridge, Mass. 13 June 1984.
10.   There are four basic categories for payers for health care costs incurred in
hospitals in Massachusetts: Medicaid, a state and federal program that pays for
the poor, blind, and disabled—those on public assistance; Medicare, a federal
program that pays for the elderly—those citizens over the age of 65; charge payers, including the private, for-profit or commercial insurance firms that pay
hospitals what they actually charge, not what the services cost, and self-pay individuals, who do not have health insurance but pay charges out-of-pocket; and
private but nonprofit insurance firms such as Blue Cross, which pay hospitals a
negotiated amount for services based on "reasonable cost." Although figures vary,
Massachusetts hospitals receive about 40 percent of their revenue from Medicare, 15 percent from Medicaid, about 25 percent from Blue Cross, and the re-
maining 15 or 20 percent from the charge and self-payers. Figures vary with
their source, but hospitals ended up charging commercial insurers between 10

and 14 percent more than they did Blue Cross. Both Blue Cross and the commercials passed these costs through to the employer-purchaser.

11. Carol Carter, "Changing the Insurance Giant: Innovations in Blue Cross Hospital Reimbursement," paper (1984):6. Ms. Carter worked for Blue Cross while she was a graduate student at the Massachusetts Institute of Technology, Cambridge, Massachusetts. This assessment, shared by most observers of Massachusetts health care politics, of Blue Cross's market share at that time is based on her access to their records. However, Blue Cross disputes that percentage. A letter from the vice president for health programs development at Blue Cross to this author, 26, January 1988, discusses their differential: "You note that we control 75 percent of the market in health insurance. This number is too high. The true number would have been about 60 percent for that period. It is currently down to about 50 percent."

12. The number of MBRT directors who were commercial insurers in 1982 was taken directly from names listed on their letterhead at the time. In a letter from John Crosier, executive director of the MBRT, to this author, 24 February 1988, he makes this point: "Six of our original members were insurance CEOs, and three of them did not sell health insurance."

13. Interview with Peter Hiam, former chair of the Massachusetts Rate Setting Commission, Boston, Mass. and Massachusetts insurance commissioner in 1984, 12 June 1984.

14. The Rate Setting Commission had approval authority over contracts between Blue Cross and the hospitals and authority in the form of a charge control system in 1982 that allowed the RSC to monitor and approve charges for the commercial insurers but not to set rates over Medicare. There were no uniform definitions of cost and no authority to force compliance from the hospitals, except to take them to court. State policy was divided on the issue of the power of the RSC to regulate hospitals. Case law said that hospitals should receive their "reasonable financial requirements," and court law said the state had the "authority to pay at a level it deemed appropriate." Blue Cross and Blue Shield had favored status because their contractual arrangements were protected by constitutional law. When the RSC tried to change price level depreciation back to historical cost depreciation and include allowances for working capital, the hospitals reacted strongly and negatively.

15. Alford, *Health Care Politics*; Murray Edelman, *The Symbolic Uses of Politics* (Urbana: University of Illinois Press, 1964); A. Twaddle and R. Hessler, "Power and Change: The Case of the Swedish Commission of Inquiry into Health and Sickness Care," *Journal of Health Politics, Policy and Law* 11:1 (1986):9–40.

16. Interview with former bureau chief of Rate Setting Commission, Boston, 12 June 1984.

17. Interview with Peter Hiam, 12 June 1984.

18. Interview with Paula Griswold, member of the health care staff for the Massachusetts Business Roundtable, in Waltham, Mass., 6 June 1984.

19. In Massachusetts the relationship between the Rate Setting Commission and Blue Cross was ambivalent. The initial methodology for Chapter 424 had been patterned after the Blue Cross contract in effect at that time; Blue Cross had been an arbiter between the hospitals and the commission in the initial negotia-

tions over the charge control system; and Blue Cross paid the salaries of 90 percent of the staff of the RSC (the commission had a staff of about 180 employees), although these employees were hired and fired by the commission itself. Commonwealth of Massachusetts, "Rate Setting Commission Annual Report for Fiscal Year 1982," 18; and Alice Sapienza, "Massachusetts Experience, Chapter 372" (Ph.D. diss., Harvard Graduate School of Business, April 22, 1983), chap. 5.

20.   Massachusetts Joint Legislative Executive Commission on Hospital Reimbursement, "Study Report, Appendix B" (Boston: Massachusetts Joint Legislative Executive Commission on Hospital Reimbursement, 17 December 1981, 15–16.

The LIAM/HIAA hospital reimbursement legislation (S. 495) called for several key points: a prospective system that would hold hospitals to approved cost and revenue limits; budget limits with the inclusion of a "productivity factor"; consistency with HA-29 and with a Medicaid or Medicare waiver; a reduction of cross-subsidies among payers; recognition of bad debt/free care costs with allocation to payers based on fair share; creation of utilization review programs to cover charge-paying patients; and implementation by 1 October 1982, with the inclusion of Medicare and Medicaid waivers. Additional information about the debate over S. 495 was drawn from an interview with Philip Caper, Kennedy School of Government, Harvard University, Cambridge, Mass., 8 June 1984.

21.   Members of the Joint Commission included nine state members (among them legislators and state bureaucrats); four business members; one labor member; three hospital representatives; one each from Blue Cross and LIAM; and no physicians or consumers. In a 18 May 1987 interview with John Crosier, staff to the business members on the commission and executive director of the MBRT at that time, he affirmed that a business member had cast the deciding vote to abolish the commission.

22.   Interview with Dennis Beatrice, staff at the Heller Graduate School of Brandeis University, Waltham, Mass., and former Massachusetts director of Medicaid in 1982, in Waltham, Mass., 11 June 1984.

23.   Interview with Gerard Desilets, staff to Massachusetts Senate Health Care Committee, Boston, 7 June 1984.

24.   Interviews with Dick Rogen, executive vice president of Blue Cross of Massachusetts, Boston, 7 June 1984, and with John Crosier, Boston, 18 May 1987.

25.   "Competition at Party's Convention," *The Boston Globe* (22 May 1984).

26.   Letter to the author from John Crosier, 24 February 1988.

27.   Interview with Steve Hegarty, vice president of finance for the Massachusetts Hospital Association, Burlington, Mass., 5 June 1984.

28.   Interview with a participant in the coalition negotiations, Boston, June 1984.

29.   Interview with Neil Foley, director of legislative affairs for the Massachusetts Medical Society, Waltham, Mass., 7 June 1984.

30.   Interview with Steve Tringale, staff to the Life Insurance Association of Massachusetts and former bureau chief at the Rate Setting Commission, Boston, 12 June 1984.

31.   Richard Knox, "Business' Push to Put a Cap on Hospital Costs," *The Boston Globe* (24 August 1982):45.

32.   Ibid.

33.   David Kinzer, internal memorandum to CEOs of the Massachusetts Hospital Association, 25 August 1982.

34.   Draft Testimony presented by the Office of Medicaid Services regarding H. 1402 to the Boston legislature, Spring 1984.

35.   Sager, "Changes in Financing Uncompensated Hospital Care in Massachusetts," 30.

36.   Massachusetts Rate Setting Commission, "Hospital Profits Increase Significantly," Press release (Boston: Massachusetts Rate Setting Commission, 21 May 1987).

37.   *Chapter 372*, Section 58: "There shall be an advisory committee to the study commission, consisting of seven members appointed by the study commission, one representing nonprofit hospital service corporations, . . . one representing companies authorized to sell accident and health insurance, . . . one person from a list of recommendations submitted by the Associated Industries of Massachusetts, one representing the interests and concerns of labor, . . . one representing the elderly, . . . one representing acute hospitals, . . . and two representing the interests and concerns of business from a list of recommendations submitted by the Massachusetts Business Roundtable."

38.   Sager, "Changes in Financing Uncompensated Hospital Care in Massachusetts," 22.

39.   Letter to the author from Karen Quigley, vice president of Blue Cross, 1 January 1988.

40.   Paul Ellwood, et al., "Chapter 372: Defining the Physician's Role. A Report to the Massachusetts Medical Society" (Excelsior, Minn.: InterStudy, 6 July 1983), 11.

41.   By late 1984, physician fees were on the agenda for regulation by the Massachusetts Department of Insurance, which had statutory authority to regulate Blue Shield payments to physicians. In Massachusetts these payments comprised the largest source of physician income. Peter Hiam, former chairman of the Rate Setting Commission under Governor King, was appointed commissioner of insurance by Governor Dukakis in 1983, and he was in charge of these 1984 hearings. A ban on balanced billing for Medicare was passed and upheld in Massachusetts courts in 1987.

42.   Interviews with staff members of the Massachusetts Rate Setting Commission, Boston, 12 June 1984. Interview with Kitty Pell, rate setting commissioner in Massachusetts, Boston, 7 June 1984.

43.   Interview with John Chapman, hospital bureau chief of the Massachusetts Rate Setting Commission, Boston, 19 May 1987.

44.   Massachusetts Hospital Association, "Double Discounting of Medicaid Case Mix in Chapter 372" (Boston, Mass.: Massachusetts Hospital Association, 1983).

45.   Richard Knox, "Dukakis Plan Seeks Free Hospital Care for 30,000," *The Boston Globe* (6 June 1984):25.

46.   Telephone interview with Richard Knox of *The Boston Globe*, 13 June 1984.

47.   Interview with state Medicaid Office staff member, Boston, 20 June 1984.

48.   Jane Stein, "Bay State Employers' Role in the Health Care Arena," *Business and Health* 3:4 (March 1986):46–49.

49.   See "Massachusetts Businesses Wrestle for Control of Medical Costs," *New*

England Business (6 September 1982); Philip Caper and David Blumenthal. "What Price Cost Control? Massachusetts' New Hospital Payment Law," *New England Journal of Medicine* 308:9 (March 1983):9; David Kinzer, "Massachusetts and California—Two Kinds of Hospital Control," *New England Journal of Medicine* 308:14 (7 April 1983):838; L. R. Gallese, "Massachusetts Law Offers New Approach to Cut Hospital Costs," *The New York Times* (13 August 1982); James Stowe, "Strengths and Weaknesses of the Massachusetts Model," *Business and Health* 1:5 (April 1984):5.

50. Kinzer, internal memorandum, 25 August 1982.

51. Interview with Gerard Desilets, 7 June 1984.

52. Interview with Willis Goldbeck, president of the Washington Business Group on Health, Washington, D.C., 14 June 1984.

53. Alford and Friedland, *Powers of Theory.*

54. Useem, *The Inner Circle.* See Useem for three organizing principles of business power that apply to this case: the upper class principle, the corporate principle, and the classwide principle.

55. Shonfield, *Modern Capitalism,* 128.

56. Richard Knox, "Mass. Enacts Health Bill," *The Boston Globe* (14 April 1988):1. Allan R. Gold, "Massachusetts Lawmakers Vote Dukakis' Health Insurance Bill," *The New York Times* (14 April 1988):4.

57. These conclusions are drawn from conversations with Professor Alan Sager of Boston University, New Orleans, Louisiana, 20 October 1987; and John Crosier, Boston, 10 September 1987.

58. Interview with Crosier, Boston, 18 May 1987.

Chapter Eight: From East to West: A Comparison of Massachusetts and California

1. See Ira Sharkansky, "Economic and Political Correlates of State Government Expenditures: General Tendencies and Deviant Cases," *Midwest Journal of Political Science* 11:2 (May 1967):173–192; Bernard Booms and James Halldorson, "The Politics of Redistribution: A Reformulation," *American Political Science Review* 67 (September 1973): 924–950.

2. Roger Friedland, Frances Fox Piven, and Robert R. Alford, "Political Conflict, Urban Structure and the Fiscal Crisis," in *Comparing Public Policies: New Concepts and Methods,* ed., Douglas Ashford (Beverly Hills, Calif.: Sage Books in Politics and Public Policy, 1977).

3. See data from "State Discretionary Policies and Services in the Medicaid, Social Services, and Supplemental Security Income Programs" (San Francisco: Aging Health Policy Center, 1983); and Robert Newcomer et al., "Policy Developments in the Medicare, Medicaid and Social Service Programs," Policy Paper No. 6 (San Francisco: Aging Health Policy Center, 1983).

4. See Linda Demkovich, "States May be Gaining in the Battle to Curb Medicaid Spending Growth," *National Journal* (18 September 1982):1584–1586; and Carroll Estes and Robert Newcomer, eds., *Fiscal Austerity and Aging* (Beverly Hills, Calif.: Sage, 1983).

5.   Michael Aiken and Robert Alford, "Community Structure and Innovation," 650–665.

6.   Raymond Wolfinger and Fred Greenstein, "Comparing Political Regions: The Case of California," *American Political Science Review* 63:1 (March 1969): 74.

7.   Written comments to the author from Clark Kerr, head of the San Francisco Business Coalition, March 1989.

8.   There were no for-profit acute care hospitals as of 1982, although there were several for-profit psychiatric hospitals.

9.   Lurie et al., "Termination from MediCal—Does it Affect Health."

10.   Sager, "Changes in Financing Uncompensated Hospital Care in Massachusetts.".

11.   Kinzer, "Massachusetts and California."

Chapter Nine: Business in the Fifty States

1.   See Karen Davis and Cathy Schoen, *Health and the War on Poverty: A Ten Year Appraisal* (Washington, D.C.: Brookings Institute, 1978); Robert Stevens and Rosemary Stevens, *Welfare Medicine in America: A Case Study of Medicaid* (New York: Free Press, 1974); Alan Spiegel and Simon Podair, *Medicaid: Lessons from National Health Insurance* (Rockville, Md.: Aspen Systems Corporation, 1975); John Palmer and Isabel Sawhill, *The Reagan Experiment* (Washington, D.C.: Urban Institute Press, 1982). When Medicare and Medicaid were passed in 1965, the emphasis of federal health policy was to increase access to care for the poor and create a single level of mainstream care for all Americans. In the 1970s as rising health care costs eroded the profit margins of large corporations, cost control became the dominant issue in the policy debate until the late 1980s. Access to care for the indigent and the lack of coverage for the working poor have placed access near the top of the agenda again by the late 1980s.

2.   See discussion in Chapter 5 about the ideological stance of the Reagan administration toward regulatory health policy change. Although the ideology of policy change in the 1980s used the language and symbols of the market approach, neither regulatory nor market approaches to policy change challenged the concept of private control over medical resources.

3.   See Chapter 5 for further discussion of the federal role as purchaser of care for Medicare and Medicaid beneficiaries. The passage of the prospective payment system for Medicare in 1983 is the most salient example of a shift in the federal role; at the state level, the California MediCal reform legislation also transformed the state from a passive financing into an active purchasing role.

4.   Theodore Lowi, *The End of Liberalism: The Second Republic of the United States* (New York: W. W. Norton, 1971).

5.   Donald Cohodes, "Where You Stand Depends on Where You Sit: Some Musings on the Regulation/Competition Dialogue," *Journal of Health Politics, Policy and Law* 7:1 (Spring 1982):54–79; Clark Havighurst, "The Current Debate Over Health Care Cost Containment Regulation: The Issues and the Interests" (Paper presented at an American Enterprise Conference, Washington,

D.C., 22 September 1983); Jack Salmon, "Who Benefits from Competition in Health Care," *Nursing Economics* 1 (September/October 1983):129–134; Paul Starr, "The Laissez-Faire Elixir," *The New Republic* (18 April 1983):19–23.

6.   Paul Ellwood and Barbara Paul, "Testing the Waters with Competition vs. Regulation," *Business and Health* 1:5 (April 1984):5–8; Eli Ginzburg, "The Grand Illusion of Competition in Health Care," *Journal of American Medical Association* 249:14 (8 April 1983):1857–1859; Bruce Owen, "Interest Group Behavior and the Political Economy of Regulation" (Paper presented at an American Enterprise Conference, Washington, D.C., 22 September 1983); Glenn Richards, "Headlines of the '80s," *Hospitals* 57:14(16 July 1983).

7.   Daniel Sigelman, "Palm Reading the Invisible Hand: A Critical Examination of the Pro-Competition Reform Proposals," *Journal of Health Politics, Policy and Law* 6:4(Winter 1982):581.

8.   Cyndee Eyster, "Special Report on Health Issues in Election Year '84: State Roundup," *FAH Review* 17:5(September/October 1984):16–35; and Barbara Paul, "State-by-State Hospital Rate Regulation Survey: Movement Toward All-Payers System and the Role of Business in Promoting All-Payers Systems," Memorandum (Excelsior, Minn.: InterStudy, 4 November 1983), 1–26.

9.   David Crozier, "State Rate-Setting: A Status Report," *Health Affairs* 1:3 (Summer 1982):66–83.

10.   Lawrence Brown as quoted in Sigelman, "Palm Reading the Invisible Hand."

11.   Average covered hospital charges per day doubled between 1981 and 1984–1985, from $346 to $627, according to a study by C. Neu and Scott Harrison, "Posthospital Care Before and After the Medicare Prospective Payment System" (Santa Monica, Calif.: Rand Corporation, March 1988), 8.

12.   Ellwood and Paul, "Testing the Waters," 6.

13.   Interview with Willis Goldbeck, president of the Washington Business Group on Health, Washington, D.C., April 1984.

14.   Kolko, *The Triumph of Conservatism*, 60.

15.   Eyster, "Special Report on Health Issues in Election Year '84;" Clearinghouse on Business Coalitions for Health Action, "Directory of Business Coalitions for Health Action" (Washington, D.C.: Chamber of Commerce of the U.S., 1984); Paul, "State-by-State Hospital Rate Regulation Survey."

16.   See Catherine McLaughlin, Wendy Zellers, and Lawrence Brown, "Health Care Coalitions: Who, What, Where, When and Why?" (Draft paper, School of Public Health, University of Michigan, 1988). Among coalitions surveyed in 1986, 58 percent of those still active had been established in 1982 and 1983.

17.   This number corresponds to the number of states with coalitions reported by hospital associations in the FAH survey, although the FAH did not include the District of Columbia. The Chamber directory did not receive any reports from eight states: Arkansas, Maine, Mississippi, Montana, New Mexico, North Dakota, South Dakota, and West Virginia. Although the FAH survey received reports from all fifty states, the FAH survey received reports from all fifty states, the FAH survey results concurred that there was no coalition activity in at least four of the Chamber's "no report" states: Mississippi, Montana, South Dakota, and West Virginia. Of the other four states, the FAH survey indicated the following

activity: in Arkansas, there were two coalitions organized but no impact to date; in Maine, activity was under way, but coalitions were not in a leadership role; in Albuquerque, New Mexico, a medical/business coalition with hospital members existed; in North Dakota, one coalition was operating, but it was not a business coalition per se. Both the FAH and Chamber data are self-reports from states and communities, but the Chamber data on coalitions were reported directly by coalition staff while the FAH relied on hospital representatives, who may not have been completely up-to-date on the status and activity of business coalitions in their states.

18.   A more recent survey of coalitions in 1986 finds active coalitions in all but five states: Alaska, Arkansas, Kentucky, Maine, and South Dakota. See McLaughlin, Zellers, and Brown, "Health Care Coalitions."

19.   Recognizing a qualitative difference between a state with one small local coalition and states with one large statewide coalition, I used the Chamber's report of statewide coalitions and moved states with one statewide coalition from the low to the medium category and states with two or three coalitions, one of which was a statewide coalition, into the high category.

20.   Nine states in the FAH survey made no mention of financial disclosure; for these states, I used the InterStudy data about rate setting to assign them to a category. Four were rate-setting states and thus had some type of mandatory disclosure; the other five states made no report, but with additional data they could be assigned to the "no financial disclosure" category.

21.   The two measures used to determine the strength of the associations between cells in this table are chi square and effect parameters, the average percentage differences in a contingency table taking account of signs. See James Coleman, *An Introduction to Mathematical Sociology* (London: Free Press of Glencoe, 1964), 194, for a more detailed description of effect parameters. In Table 9.2, the effect parameter is calculated in the following way, determined by the expected direction of the change: 11 is subtracted from 12, 12 from 50, then 44 from 56, and 13 from 44. These numbers are added together and divided by four to reach an effect parameter of plus 21. In this case all four numbers are positive because the direction of change is as predicted. However, if any one of them had been negative, that number would have been subtracted instead of added. Effect parameters of between 0 and 7 are considered to range from no effect to a slight effect; between 8 and 15 indicates a moderate effect; and over 15 is a strong effect. Chi squares of under 5 are considered to show little association, and chi squares over 10 show a stronger association.

22.   Linda Bergthold, "Business and the Politics of Health Policy Change" (Ph.D. diss., University of California, Santa Cruz, 1985), 519–625.

23.   Ibid.

24.   McLaughlin, Zellers, and Brown, "Health Care Coalitions."

25.   The McLaughlin, Zellers, and Brown study also concluded that education, data collection, and legislative advocacy were lower priorities for employer-only coalitions than benefit plan design or alternative delivery system development.

Chapter Ten: Purchasing Alliances in Health

1. The conditions under which a community might be ready for health system change are taken from remarks made by Bruce Spitz, director of the Pew Associates Program and associate director of the Bigel Institute of Health Policy Studies at Brandeis University, Waltham, Mass (Remarks, conference, cosponsored by the Washington Business Group on Health and the National Governors' Association, Boulder, Colorado, 16–17 January 1984).

For more information from the literature on policy innovation, see Walker, "The Diffusion of Innovations Among American States," 880–900; Aiken and Alford, "Community Structure and Innovation," 650–665; Robert Crain, "Fluoridation: The Diffusion of an Innovation Among Cities," *Social Forces* 44:4 (June 1966):467–476; and Elihu Katz, Martin Levi, and Herbert Hamilton, "Traditions of Research in the Diffusion of Innovations," *American Sociological Review* 57 (1963):237-252.

2. Jon Gabel et al. "The Changing World of Group Health Insurance," *Health Affairs* 7:3 (Summer 1988):64; and Simon Francis, "U.S. Industrial Outlook, 1989: Health Services" (Washington, D.C.: U.S. Department of Commerce January 1989), as quoted in *Medical Benefits* 6:3(15 February 1989):1–2.

3. Sheldon Wolin, "The New Public Philosophy," *democracy*(October 1981):35. Note: By the end of the 1980s, there are signs that merely addressing costs will be insufficient to solve the policy problems. A lack of access to medical coverage has become both a cost and a distribution issue.

4. Havighurst, "The Changing Locus of Decision Making in the Health Care Sector," 724.

5. Wolin, "New Public Philosophy," 35.

6. Burnett as quoted in Iglehart, "Big Business and Health Care in the Heartland."

7. Havighurst, "The Changing Locus of Decision Making in the Health Care Sector," 718.

8. See Starr, *The Social Transformation of American Medicine.*

9. Jeff Goldsmith, "Competition's Impact: A Report from the Front," Commentary in *Health Affairs* 7:3 (Summer 1988):166.

10. Interview with Walter McNerney, former president of Blue Cross, Chicago, 3 March 1988.

11. Telephone interview with Bert Seidman of the AFL-CIO, 29 January 1988.

12. Clarence Stone, *Economic Growth and Neighborhood Discontent* (Chapel Hill: N.C. University of North Carolina Press, 1976.

13. Nolan, "Political Surfing When Issues Break," 73.

14. Doug Lefton, "Behind-Scenes Story of Coalition Defeat," *American Medical News* (29 March 1985):9.

15. Brown and McLaughlin, " 'May the Third Force Be with You.' "

16. For further discussion, see Carroll Estes, Elizabeth A. Binney, and Linda Bergthold, "The Delegitimation of the Nonprofit Sector: The Role of Ideology and Public Policy," in *Looking Forward to the Year 2000: Public Policy and Philanthropy*, Spring Research Forum, Working Papers (New York: The Independent Sector, 17 March 1988), 498–516. See also Theodore Marmor, Mark

Schlesinger, and R. W. Smithey, "Nonprofit Organizations and Health Care," in *The Nonprofit Sector: A Research Handbook*, ed. W. W. Powell, 221–239 (New Haven: Yale University Press, 1987); Susan Ostrander, S. Langton, and J. Von Til, *The Shifting Debate* (New Brunswick, N.J.: Transaction Books, 1987); and W. A. Nielsen, *The Endangered Sector* (New York: Columbia University Press, 1979).

17.   Telephone interview with Bert Seidman.

18.   Useem, *The Inner Circle*, 17.

19.   Evans, "Finding the Levers, Finding the Courage," 603.

20.   See McConnell, *Private Power and American Democracy*; Shonfield, *Modern Capitalism*; Peter Hall, "Economic Planning and the State: The Evolution of Economic Challenge and Political Response in France," in *Political Power and Social Theory*, ed. Maurice Zeitlin, 175–214 (Greenwich, Conn.: JAI Press, 1982); and Lindblom, *Politics and Markets*.

21.   Bruce Keppel, "Arizona in Battle Over Health Care," *Los Angeles Times* (8 May 1984), Part IV:1.

22.   Brown and McLaughlin, " 'May the Third Force Be with You,' " 13.

23.   Interview with Walter McNerney.

24.   Interview with James Sammons, M.D., executive vice president of the AMA, Chicago, 3 March 1988.

25.   Interview with Alexander Williams, vice president of the AHA, Chicago, 2 March 1988.

26.   "There's Still No Cure for Exploding Health Care Costs," *Business Week* (22 September 1986):16; Neu and Harrison, *Posthospital Care Before and After the Medicare Prospective Payment System*; and Michael Pollock and Vicky Cahan, "Why Health Care Costs are Having a Relapse," *Business Week* (12 May 1986):34; Uwe Reinhardt, "The Real Numbers Don't Add Up to Health-Cost Savings," as quoted in *Medical Benefits* (30 September 1987):6; Michael Booth, "Colorado Firms Unite to Bargain for Lower Health Care Fees," *Healthweek* (14 March 1988):17; and A. Foster Higgins, "Health Care Benefit Survey, 1988," as quoted in *Medical Benefits* 6:4 (28 February 1989):1–2.

27.   Jeffrey C. Goldsmith as quoted in Pollock and Cahan, "Why Health Care Costs Are Having a Relapse," 34.

28.   "Benefits and the Bottom Line" (Report on Health Care Costs, Kansas City, Missouri, May 1988), as quoted in "Mercer in the News" (May/June 1988), a compendium of articles and quotes compiled by Mercer Meidinger Hansen, New York.

29.   Hennessy, "A Completely New Way to Purchase Medical Benefits."

30.   A study by Mercer Meidinger Hansen, Inc., and the Mid-America Coalition, as quoted in "Benefits and the Bottom Line," 68.

31.   Interview with Walter McNerney.

32.   Hennessey, "A Completely New Way to Purchase Medical Benefits."

33.   Michael Booth, "Colorado Firms Unite to Bargain," 34.

34.   Jeff Goldsmith, "Competition's Impact," 162.

35.   Ibid., 163.

Bibliography

Aiken, Michael, and Robert R. Alford. "Community Structure and Innovation: The Case of Urban Renewal." *American Sociological Review* 35 (August 1970):650–665.

Alford, Robert R. *Bureaucracy and Participation: Political Culture in Four Wisconsin Cities.* Chicago: Rand McNally, 1969.

――――. *Health Care Politics: Ideological and Interest Group Barriers to Reform.* Chicago: University of Chicago Press, 1975.

Alford, Robert R., and Roger Friedland. "Political Participation in Public Policy." *Annual Review of Sociology* 1 (1975):429–479.

――――. *Powers of Theory, Capitalism, The State, and Democracy.* New York: Cambridge University Press, 1985.

Anton, Thomas. "The Regional Distribution of Federal Expenditures, 1971–1980." *National Tax Journal* 36:4 (December 1983):429–442.

Bachrach, Peter, and Morton Baratz. "The Two Faces of Power." *American Political Science Review* 56 (1962):947–952.

Banks, Louis. "Taking on the Hostile Media." *Harvard Business Review* 56 (March/April 1978):123–130.

Bauer, Raymond, Ithiel de Sola Pool, and Lewis A. Dexter. *American Business and Public Policy.* 2d ed. New York: Atherton, 1972.

Bell, Colin, and Howard Newby, eds. *Doing Sociological Research.* London: George Allen and Unwin, 1977.

Bergthold, Linda. "Business and the Pushcart Vendors in an Age of Supermarkets." *International Journal of Health Services* 17:1 (1987):7–26.

――――. "The Business Community as a Promoter of Change." *Business and Health* 3:3 (January/February 1986):39–41.

――――. "Crabs in a Bucket: The Politics of Health Care Reform in California." *Journal of Health Politics, Policy and Law* 9:2 (Summer 1984):203–222.

――――. "Purchasing Power: Business and Health Policy Change in Massachusetts." *Journal of Health Politics, Policy and Law* 13:3 (Fall 1988):425–451.

Berliner, Howard. "A Larger Perspective on the Flexner Report." *International Journal of Health Services* 5:4 (1975):513–592.

———. *A System of Scientific Medicine: Philanthropic Foundations in the Flexner Era*. New York: Tavistock, 1985.

Blalock, Hubert M., Jr. *Social Statistics*. New York: McGraw-Hill, 1960.

Blum, Henrik. *Expanding Health Care Horizons*. 2d ed. Oakland: Third Party Publishing Company, 1983.

Brown, E. R. *Rockefeller Medicine Men: Medicine and Capitalism in America*. Berkeley: University of California Press, 1979.

Brown, Lawrence D. "Competition and Health Care Cost Competition: Cautions and Conjectures." *Milbank Memorial Fund Quarterly/Health and Society* 59 (Spring 1981):179.

———. "Introduction to a Decade of Transition." *Journal of Health Politics, Policy and Law* 11:4 (1986):569–583.

———. *New Policies, New Politics: Government's Response to Government's Growth*. Washington, D.C.: Brookings Institution, 1983.

———. *Politics and Health Care Organizations: HMOs as Federal Policy*. Washington, D.C.: Brookings Institution, 1983.

———. "Technocratic Corporatism and Administrative Reform in Medicare." *Journal of Health Politics, Policy and Law* 10:3 (Fall 1985):579–599.

Brown, Lawrence, and Catherine McLaughlin. "'May the Third Force Be With You': Community Programs for Affordable Health Care." In *Advances in Health Economics and Health Services Research*, Vol. 8, ed. Richard Scheffler and L. F. Rossiter. Greenwich, Conn.: JAI Press, 1988.

Burgess, Robert. *In the Field: An Introduction to Field Research*. London: George Allen and Unwin, 1984.

Business Roundtable Task Force on Health. "Corporate Health Care Cost Management and Private Sector Initiatives, 1984 Survey." Washington, D.C.: Business Roundtable, 1984.

Cain, Carol. "Coalitions Continue Attack on Health Costs." *Business Insurance* (2 May 1983):21–25.

Califano, Joseph. *America's Health Care Revolution*. New York: Random House, 1986.

Caper, Phillip, and David Blumenthal. "What Price Cost Control? Massachusetts' New Hospital Payment Law." *New England Journal of Medicine* 308:9 (3 May 1983):542–544.

Cawson, Alan. *Corporatism and Political Theory*. New York: Basil Blackwell, 1986.

Clark, Terry. "Community Structure, Decision-Making, Budget Expenditures, and Renewal in 51 American Communities." *American Sociological Review* 33 (1968):576–593.

Coleman, James S. *Introduction to Mathematical Sociology*. London: Free Press of Glencoe, 1964.

Cohen, Joshua, and Joel Rogers. *On Democracy: Toward a Transformation of American Society*. New York: Penguin Books, 1983.

Cohen, Richard. "The Business Lobby Discovers That in Unity There is Strength." *National Journal* (28 June 1980):1050–1053.

Cohen, Stephen, and Charles Goldfinger. "From Permacrisis to Real Crisis in French Social Security: The Limits to Normal Politics." In *Stress and Contradiction in Modern Capitalism,* ed. Leon Lindberg et al., 57–99. Lexington, Mass.: D. C. Heath, 1975.

Cohodes, Donald. "Where You Stand Depends On Where You Sit: Some Musings on the Regulation/Competition Dialogue." *Journal of Health Politics, Policy and Law* 7:1 (Spring 1982):54–79.

Committee for Economic Development. "Building a National Health Care System." New York: Committee for Economic Development, April 1973.

Committee on the Costs of Medical Care. *Medical Care for the American People: The Final Report of the Committee on the Costs of Medical Care.* Chicago: University of Chicago Press, 1932.

Council on Wage and Price Stability. *The Problem of Rising Health Care Costs.* Washington, D.C.: U.S. Government Printing Office, 26 April 1976.

Crain, Robert. "Fluoridation: The Diffusion of an Innovation Among Cities." *Social Forces* 44:4 (June 1966):467–476.

Crenson, Matthew. *The Un-Politics of Air Pollution: A Study of Non-Decision Making in the Cities.* Baltimore: John Hopkins University Press, 1971.

Crozier, David. "State Rate-Setting: A Status Report." *Health Affairs* 1:3 (Summer 1982):66–83.

Dahl, Robert. "The Concept of Power." In *Political Power: A Reader in Theory and Research,* ed. Roderick Bell, David M. Edwards, R. Harrison Wagner. New York: Free Press, 1969.

———. *Who Governs? Power and Democracy in an American City.* New Haven, Conn.: Yale University Press, 1961.

Davis, Karen, and Cathy Schoen. *Health and the War on Poverty: A Ten Year Appraisal.* Washington, D.C.: Brookings Institution, 1978.

Demkovich, Linda. "Business as a Health Care Consumer is Paying Heed to the Bottom Line." *National Journal* (24 May 1980):851–854.

———. "Health Insurers Favor Budget Cutting—But Not If It Means They Must Pay More." *National Journal* (21 November 1981):2068–2070.

———. "States May Be Gaining in the Battle to Curb Medicaid Spending Growth." *National Journal* (18 September 1982):1584–1586.

Domhoff, G. William. *The Higher Circles: The Governing Class in America.* New York: Random House, 1970.

———. *The Powers That Be: Processes of Ruling Class Domination in America.* New York: Random House, 1979.

———. *Who Rules America?* Englewood Cliffs, N.J.: Prentice-Hall, 1967.

———. *Who Rules America Now? A View for the '80s.* New York: Simon and Schuster, 1983.

Dunham, Andrew B., and James Morone. *The Politics of Innovation: The Evolution of DRG Rate Regulation in New Jersey.* Princeton, N.J.: Health Research and Educational Trust, 1983.

Dunlop, John, ed. *Business and Public Policy.* Cambridge, Mass.: Harvard University Press, 1980.

Dye, Thomas R. *Politics, Economics and the Public: Policy Outcomes in the American States.* Chicago: Rand-McNally, 1966.

_____. *Understanding Public Policy.* Englewood Cliffs, N.J.: Prentice-Hall, 1972.

_____. *Who's Running America?* Englewood Cliffs, N.J.: Prentice-Hall, 1976.

Easton, David. *A Systems Analysis of Political Life.* New York: Wiley and Sons, 1965.

Edelman, Murray. *The Symbolic Uses of Politics.* Urbana: University of Illinois Press, 1985.

Egdahl, Richard. "Health Cost Management at the Community Level: Doctors, Hospitals and Industry." *Health Affairs* 2:3 (Fall 1983):113–125.

_____. "Should We Shrink the Health Care System?" *Harvard Business Review* (January/February 1984):125–130.

Ellwood, Paul, and Barbara Paul. "Testing the Waters with Competition vs. Regulation." *Business and Health* 1:5 (April 1984):5–8.

Epstein, Edwin M. *The Corporation in American Politics.* Englewood Cliffs, N.J.: Prentice-Hall, 1969.

Estes, Carroll L. *The Aging Enterprise.* San Francisco: Jossey-Bass, 1979.

_____. *The Decision Makers.* Dallas: Southern Methodist University Press, 1963.

Estes, Carroll, and Robert J. Newcomer, eds. *Fiscal Austerity and Aging.* Beverly Hills, Calif.: Sage, 1983.

Falk, Marilyn, and Eileen Tell. "Private Sector Initiatives: What Makes Them Work?" *Business and Health* 1:4 (March 1984):27–31.

Feder, Judith. *Medicare: The Politics of Federal Hospital Insurance.* Lexington, Mass.: Lexington Books, 1977.

Fenton, John H., and Donald Chamberlayne. "The Literature Dealing with the Relationships Between Political Processes, Socio-Economic Conditions, and Public Policies in the American States: A Bibliographic Essay." *Polity* 1 (Spring 1969):388–394.

Flexner, Abraham. *Medical Education in the United States and Canada,* Bulletin No. 4. New York: Carnegie Foundation for the Advancement of Teaching, 1910.

Fox, Peter, Willis B. Goldbeck, and Jacob J. Spies, eds. *Health Care Cost Management.* Ann Arbor, Mich.: Health Administration Press, 1984).

Friedland, Roger. "Central City Fiscal Strains: The Public Costs of Private Growth." *International Journal of Urban and Regional Research* 5:3 (September 1981):356–376.

_____. "The Local Economy of Political Power: Participation, Organization and Dominance." *Pacific Sociological Review* 24:2 (April 1981):139–174.

Friedland, Roger, and Donald Palmer. "Park Place and Main Street: Business and the Urban Power Structure." *Annual Review of Sociology* 10 (1984): 395–416.

Friedland, Roger, Frances Fox Piven, and Robert R. Alford. "Political Conflict, Urban Structure, and the Fiscal Crisis." In *Comparing Public Policies: New Concepts and Methods,* ed. Douglas Ashford. 197–225. Beverly Hills, Calif.: Sage, 1977.

Gerber, Paul. "How Health Care Coalitions Will Affect Your Practice." *Physician's Management* (February 1986):200–215.

Giddens, Anthony. *Central Problems in Social Theory: Action, Structure and Contradiction in Social Analysis.* London: Macmillan, 1979.

Ginsburg, Paul, and Frank Sloan. "Hospital Cost-Shifting." *New England Journal of Medicine* 310:14 (5 April 1984):893–895.

Ginzberg, Eli. "The Grand Illusion of Competition in Health Care." *Journal of American Medical Association* 249:14 (8 April 1983):1857–1859.

———. *The Limits of Health Reform: The Search for Realism.* New York: Basic Books, 1977.

Gottlieb, Symond. "Ensuring Access to Health Care: What Communities Can Do to Make a Difference Through Private Sector Coalitions." *Inquiry* 23 (Fall 1986):322–329.

Greenstein, Fred, and Nelson Polsby. *Policies and Policymaking: Handbook of Political Science.* Vol. 6. Reading, Mass.: Addison-Wesley, 1975.

Hawley, Willis, and Frederick Wirt. *The Search for Community Power.* Englewood Cliffs, N.J.: Prentice-Hall, 1968.

Henderson, Robert R., and J. Joel May. "The Business Community Looks at DRG-Based Hospital Reimbursement." *Health Affairs* 2:1 (Spring 1983): 38–49.

Herzlinger, Regina. "How Companies Tackle Health Care Costs, Part II." *Harvard Business Review* 63:5 (September–October 1985):120.

Hiatt, Howard. "The Coming of Corporate Medicine." *Harvard Business Review* 62 (January/February 1984):6–10.

Hicks, Alexander, Roger Friedland, and Edwin Johnson. "Class Power and State Policy: The Case of Large Business Corporations, Unions and Governmental Redistribution in the American States." *American Political Science Review* 43:3 (June 1978):302–316.

Hofferbert, Richard. "Classification of American State Party Systems." *Journal of Politics* (1964):550–567.

———. "Elite Influence in State Policy Formation. A Model for Comparative Inquiry." *Polity* 2:3 (Spring 1970):316–344.

———. "The Relation Between Public Policy and Some Structural and Environmental Variables in the American States." *American Political Science Review* 60 (March 1966):73–82.

Holland, Daniel, and Stewart Myers. "Profitability and Capital Costs for Manufacturing Corporations and All Nonfinancial Corporations." *American Economic Review* 70 (1980):320–325.

Hunter, Floyd. *Community Power Structure.* Chapel Hill: University of North Carolina Press, 1953.

Huntington, Samuel. *American Politics: The Promise of Disharmony.* Cambridge, Mass.: Belknap Press, 1981.

Hyman, Herbert Harvey, ed. *The Politics of Health Care: Nine Case Studies of Innovative Planning in New York City.* New York: Praeger, 1973.

Igelhart, John. "Drawing the Lines for the Debate on Competition." *The New England Journal of Medicine* 305:5 (30 July 1981):292.

_____. "Health Care and American Business." *New England Journal of Medicine* 306 (14 January 1982):120–124.

Jaeger, Jon, ed. *Private Sector Coalitions: A Fourth Party in Health Care?* Durham, N.C.: Duke University Press, 1983.

Jenkins, W. I. *Policy Analysis: A Political and Organisational Perspective.* London: Martin Robertson, 1978.

Katz, Elihu, Martin Levi, and Herbert Hamilton. "Traditions of Research in the Diffusion of Innovations." *American Sociological Review* 28 (1963):237–252.

Kaufman, Herbert. "The Political Ingredient of Public Health Services: A Neglected Area of Research." *Milbank Memorial Fund Quarterly* 44 (October 1966):30–31.

Kinzer, David. "Massachusetts and California: Two Kinds of Hospital Cost Control." *New England Journal of Medicine* 308:14 (7 April 1983):838–841.

Kirkland, Richard, Jr. "Fat Days for the Chamber of Commerce." *Fortune* (21 September 1981):144–157.

Kolko, Gabriel. *The Triumph of Conservatism: A Reinterpretation of American History, 1900–1916.* 2d ed. New York: Free Press, 1967.

Kuznets, Simon. "Long Swings in the Growth of Population and in Related Economic Variables." *Proceedings of the American Philosophical Society* (February 1958):25–52.

Lanning, Joyce, and Myron D. Fottler. "Coalitions for Health Care: New Interorganizational Relations Affecting the Delivery of Health Care." Paper presented at the Academy of Management, January 1984.

Larson, Magali Sarfatti. *The Rise of Professionalism.* Berkeley: University of California Press, 1977.

Law, Sylvia. *Blue Cross: What Went Wrong?* New Haven, Conn.: Yale University Press, 1974.

Lehmbruch, Gerhard. "Liberal Corporatism and Party Government. *Comparative Political Studies* 10:1 (April 1977):91–127.

Levitan, Sar A., and Martha Cooper. *Business Lobbies, The Public Good and the Bottom Line.* Baltimore, Md.: Johns Hopkins University Press, 1984.

Lincoln, J. R. "Organizational Dominance and Community Power Structure." In *Power, Paradigms and Community Research,* ed. R. Liebert and A. Imershein, 19–50. Beverly Hills, Calif.: Sage, 1977.

Lindberg, Leon, Robert Alford, Colin Crouch, and Claus Offe. *Stress and Contradiction in Modern Capitalism.* Lexington, Mass.: D. C. Heath, 1975.

Lindblom, Charles E. *The Policy-Making Process.* Englewood Cliffs, N.J.: Prentice-Hall, 1968.

_____. *Politics and Markets: The World's Political-Economic Systems.* New York: Basic Books, 1977.

Lipset, Seymour M. *Political Man: The Social Bases of Politics.* Baltimore, Md.: Johns Hopkins University Press, 1981.

Lockard, Duane. *New England State Politics.* Princeton, N.J.: Princeton University Press, 1959.

Lowi, Theodore. *The End of Liberalism: The Second Republic of the United States.* New York: W. W. Norton, 1979.

Lukes, Steven. *Power: A Radical View.* London: Macmillan, 1974.

Lurie, Nicole, Nancy Ward, Martin Shapiro, and Robert Brook. "Termination from Medi-Cal—Does It Affect Health?" *New England Journal of Medicine* 311:7 (16 August 1984):480–484.

Lynk, William. "Reglation and Competition: An Examination of the Consumer Choice Health Plans." *Journal of Health Politics, Policy and Law* 6:4 (Winter 1982):625–637.

McConnell, Grant. *Private Power and American Democracy*. New York: Alfred A. Knopf, 1967.

Marmor, Theodore. *Political Analysis and American Medical Care*. (Cambridge: Cambridge University Press, 1983.

———. *The Politics of Medicare*. Chicago: Aldine Publishing Company, 1973.

Marmor, Theodore, Mark Schlesinger, and R. W. Smithey. "Nonprofit Organizations and Health Care." In *The Nonprofit Sector: A Research Handbook*, ed. W. W. Powell, 221–239. New Haven: Yale University Press, 1987.

Marshall, D. R. *The Politics of Participation in Poverty: A Case Study of the Board of Economic and Youth Opportunities Agency of Greater Los Angeles*. Berkeley: University of California Press, 1971.

Melia, Edward, Leonard Aucoin, Leonard Duhl, Patsy Kurokawa. "Competition in the Health Care Marketplace, A Beginning in California." *New England Journal of Medicine* 308:13 (31 March 1983):788–792.

Meyer, Jack, ed. *Market Reforms in Health Care*. Washington, D.C.: American Enterprise Institute, 1983.

Meyerhoff, Allen, and David A. Crozier. "Health Care Coalitions: The Evolution of a Movement." *Health Affairs* 3:1 (Spring 1984):120–129.

Miller, Irwin. "Intrepreneurship: A Community Coalition Approach to Health Care Reform." *Inquiry* 24 (Fall 1987):266–275.

Mills, Charles Wright. *The Sociological Imagination*. New York: Oxford University Press, 1959.

Mills, Gregory B., and John L. Palmer. *Federal Budget Policy in the 1980s*. Washington, D.C.: Urban Institute Press, 1984.

Morone, James, and Andrew Dunham. "The Waning of Professional Dominance: DRGs and the Hospitals." *Health Affairs* 2:3 (Fall 1983):73–87.

Nadel, Mark N. *Corporations and Political Accountability*. Lexington, Mass.: D. C. Heath, 1976.

Navarro, Vicente, ed. *Health and Medical Care in the U.S.: A Critical Analysis*. Farmingdale, N.Y.: Baywood Publishing Company, 1975.

———. "Political Power, The State and Their Implications in Medicine." *The Review of Radical Political Economics* 9:1 (Spring 1977):61–80.

O'Connor, James. *Accumulation Crisis*. Oxford, Eng.: Basil Blackwell, 1984.

———. *The Fiscal Crisis of the State*. New York: St. Martins Press, 1973.

Offe, Claus. "The Theory of the Capitalist State and the Problem of Policy Formation." In *Stress and Contradiction in Modern Capitalism*, ed. Leon Lindberg et al., 125–145. Lexington, Mass.: D. C. Heath, 1975.

Offe, Claus, and Volker Ronge. "Theses on the Theory of the State." In *Class, Power and Conflict,* ed. Anthony Giddens and David Held, 139–147. Berkeley: University of California Press, 1982.

Palmer, John, and Isabel Sawhill. *The Reagan Experiment.* Washington, D.C.: Urban Institute Press, 1982.

Pelligrini, R. J., and C. H. Coates. "Absentee-Owned Corporations and Community Power Structure." *American Journal of Sociology* 61 (1956):413–419.

Perrow, Charles. *Complex Organizations.* New York: Random House, 1979.

Perrucci, R., and Marc Pilisuk. "Leaders and Ruling Elites: The Interorganizational Basis of Community Power." *American Sociological Review* 36 (1970):1040–1057.

Petersdorf, Robert. "Progress Report on Hospital Cost Control in California: More Regulation Than Competition." *New England Journal of Medicine* 309:4 (28 July 1983):254–256.

Piven, Frances Fox, and Richard Cloward. *The New Class War: Reagan's Attack on the Welfare State.* New York: Pantheon Books, 1982.

Pollitt, Christopher. "Corporate Rationalization of American Health Care: A Visitor's Appraisal." *Journal of Health Politics, Policy and Law* 7:1 (Spring 1982): 227–253.

Polsby, Nelson W. *Community Power and Political Theory.* New Haven: Yale University Press, 1963.

Reagan, Michael D. "The Seven Fallacies of Business in Politics." *Harvard Business Review* 38:2 (March/April 1960):60–68.

Reisler, Mark. "Business in Richmond Attacks Health Care Costs." *Harvard Business Review* 63:1 (January/February 1985):145–155.

Relman, Arnold. "Investor-Owned Hospitals and Health Care Costs." *New England Journal of Medicine* 309:6 (11 August 1983):370–372.

"A Report on Coalitions to Contain Health Care Costs." Washington, D.C.: Government Research Corporation, 1979.

Rose, Arnold. *The Power Structure: Political Process in American Society.* London: Oxford University Press, 1967.

Rowbottom, Ralph. *Social Analysis.* London: Heinemann, 1977.

Salmon, Jack. "Corporate Attempts to Reorganize the American Health Care System." Ph.D. diss., Cornell University, 1978.

———. "The Health Maintenance Organization Strategy: A Corporate Takeover of Health Services Delivery." *International Journal of Health Services* 5:4 (1975):609–669.

———. "Who Benefits from Competition in Health Care?" *Nursing Economics* 1 (September/October 1983):129–134.

Salzman, Hal. "The Massachusetts Business Roundtable." A case study in *Who Rules Boston?* Ed. Boston Urban Study Group. Boston: Institute for Democratic Socialism, 1984.

Sapolsky, Harvey, Drew Altman, Richard Green, and Judith Moore. "Corporate Attitudes Toward Health Care Costs." *Milbank Memorial Fund Quarterly/Health and Society* 59:4 (1981):560–585.

Schattschneider, E. E. *The Semisovereign People: A Realist's View of Democracy in America.* Hinsdale, Ill.: Dryden Press, 1960.

Scheffler, Richard, and L. F. Rossiter, eds. *Advances in Health Economics and Health Services Research,* Vol. 8. Greenwich, Conn.: JAI Press, 1988.

Schlesigner, Mark. "The Rise of Proprietary Health Care." *Business and Health* 2:3 (January/February 1985):7–12.

Schmitter, P. C. "Still the Century of Corporatism?" *Review of Politics* 36 (1974): 85–131.

Schmitter, Phillippe, and Gerhard Lehmbruch, eds. *Trends Towards Corporatist Intermediation.* Beverly Hills, Calif.: Sage, 1979.

Seidelman, Raymond M. "Pluralist Heaven's Dissenting Angels: Corporatism in the American Political Economy." In *The Political Economy of Public Policy,* 59–73. Beverly Hills, Calif.: Sage, 1982.

Selznick, Philip. *TVA and the Grass Roots.* Berkeley: University of California Press, 1949.

Shapiro, Irving. *America's Third Revolution: Public Interest and the Private Role.* New York: Harper & Row, 1984.

———. "Learning to Set a Limit on Health Care." *Business Week* (14 February 1983).

Sharkansky, Ira. "Economic and Political Correlates of State Government Expenditures: General Tendencies and Deviant Cases." *Midwest Journal of Political Science* 11:2 (May 1967):173–192.

———. "Government Expenditures and Public Services in the American States." *American Political Science Review* 61 (1967):1066–1077.

Sharkansky, Ira, and Richard Hofferbert. "Dimensions of State Politics, Economics and Public Policy." *American Political Science Review* 63 (1969):867–879.

Shonfield, Andrew. *Modern Capitalism: The Changing Balance of Public and Private Power.* New York: Oxford University Press, 1969.

Sigelman, Daniel W. "Palm-Reading the Invisible Hand: A Critical Examination of the Pro-Competition Reform Proposals." *Journal of Health Politics, Policy and Law* 6:4 (Winter 1982):578–619.

Silk, Leonard, and David Vogel. *Ethics and Profits: The Crisis of Confidence in American Business.* New York: Simon and Schuster, 1976.

Skocpol, Theda. "Political Response to the Capitalist Crisis: Neo-Marxist Theories of the State and the Case of the New Deal." *Politics and Society* 10:2 (1980):155–201.

Slavin, Peter. "The Business Roundtable: New Lobbying Arm of Big Business." *Business and Society Review* (Winter 1975–1976):28–32.

Smelser, Neil J. *Comparative Methods in the Social Sciences.* Englewood Cliffs, N.J.: Prentice-Hall, 1976.

Spiegel, Alan, and Simon Podair. *Medicaid: Lessons From National Health Insurance.* Rockville, Md.: Aspen Systems Corporation, 1975.

Starr, Paul. "Controlling Medical Costs Through Countervailing Power." *Working Papers* (Summer 1977):10–11, 97–98.

———. "The Laissez-Faire Elixir." *The New Republic.* (18 April 1983): 19–23.

———. *The Social Transformation of American Medicine.* New York: Basic Books, 1982.

Stein, Jane. "New Goals for Business Coalitions." *Business and Health* 2:7 (June 1985):42–45.

Stevens, Robert, and Rosemary Stevens. *Welfare Medicine in America: A Case Study of Medicaid.* New York: Free Press, 1974.

Stone, Clarence. *Economic Growth and Neighborhood Discontent.* Chapel Hill: University of North Carolina Press, 1976.

———. "Systemic Power in Community Decision-Making: A Restatement for Stratification Theory." *American Political Science Review* 74:4 (1980): 978–990.

Streeck, Wolfgang, and P. C. Schmitter. *Private Interest Government, Beyond Market and State.* London: Sage, 1985.

Tell, Eileen, Marilyn Falik, and Peter D. Fox. "Private-Sector Health Care Initiatives: A Comparative Perspective from Four Communities." *Milbank Memorial Fund Quarterly/Health and Society* 62:3 (1984):357–379.

Thompson, Frank. *Health Policy and the Bureaucracy.* Cambridge, Mass.: MIT Press, 1981.

Truman, David. *The Governmental Process: Political Interests and Public Opinion.* New York: Alfred A. Knopf, 1971.

Turk, Herman. "Interorganizational Networks in Urban Society: Initial Perspectives and Comparative Research." *American Sociological Review* 35:1 (February 1970):1–19.

Twaddle, A., and R. Hessler. "Power and Change: The Case of the Swedish Commission of Inquiry into Health and Sickness Care." *Journal of Health Politics, Policy and Law* 11:1 (1986):9–40.

Useem, Michael. *The Inner Circle: Large Corporations and the Rise of Business Political Activity in the U.S. and U.K.* New York: Oxford University Press, 1984.

———. "Which Business Leaders Help Govern." In *Power Structure Research*, ed. G. William Domhoff, 199–227. Beverly Hills, Calif.: Sage, 1980.

Walker, Jack. "The Diffusion of Innovations Among the American States." *American Political Science Review* 63:3 (September 1969):880–900.

Walton, John. "The Structural Bases of Political Change in Urban Communities." *Sociological Inquiry* 43:3 (1973):174–206.

———. "The Vertical Axis of Community Organization and the Structure of Power." *Social Science Quarterly* 48 (1967):353–368.

Weinstein, James. *The Corporate Ideal in the Liberal State: 1900–1918.* Boston: Beacon Press, 1968.

Werntz, Raymond, and Miller, Jeffrey. "Illinois Looks to Data Gathering Council to Spur Competitive Cost Reform." *Business and Health* 2:3 (January/February 1985):50–53.

Wheaton, William. "Interstate Differences in the Level of Business Taxation." *National Tax Journal* 36:1 (March 1983):81–92.

Whitt, Alan J. "Toward a Class-Dialectic Model of Power: An Empirical Assessment of Three Competing Models of Political Power." *American Sociological Review* 44 (1979):81–100.

———. *Urban Elites and Mass Transportation: The Dialectics of Power.* Princeton, N.J.: Princeton University Press, 1982.

Wikler, Daniel. "Forming an Ethical Response to For-Profit Health Care." *Business and Health* 2:3 (January/February 1985):25–29.

Wilson, Graham K. *Business and Politics: A Comparative Introduction*. London: Macmillan, 1985.

Wolfinger, Raymond E., and Greenstein, Fred I. "Comparing Political Regions: The Case of California." *American Political Science Review* 63:1 (March 1969):74–86.

York, Chris. "Business and 'the Common'." *Inquiry* 23 (Fall 1986):299–307.

Zeitlin, Maurice, ed. *Political Power and Social Theory: A Research Annual*. Vol. 2. Greenwich, Conn.: JAI Press, 1981.

Index

37.00